Dear Kathy –

I heard this woman speak on public radio this spring. I hope you enjoy this. Happy Birthday 2000 and best wishes for a fulfilling year ahead.

Your old friend

Ann

Self-Nurture

VIKING

75 years

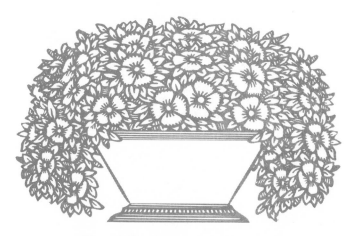

Self-Nurture

Learning to Care for Yourself

as Effectively as You Care

for Everyone Else

ALICE D. DOMAR, PH.D.,

AND HENRY DREHER

VIKING

VIKING
Published by the Penguin Group
Penguin Putnam Inc., 375 Hudson Street,
New York, New York 10014, U.S.A.
Penguin Books Ltd, 27 Wrights Lane, London W8 5TZ, England
Penguin Books Australia Ltd, Ringwood, Victoria, Australia
Penguin Books Canada Ltd, 10 Alcorn Avenue,
Toronto, Ontario, Canada M4V 3B2
Penguin Books (N.Z.) Ltd, 182–190 Wairau Road,
Auckland 10, New Zealand

Penguin Books Ltd, Registered Offices:
Harmondsworth, Middlesex, England

First published in 2000 by Viking Penguin,
a member of Penguin Putnam Inc.

1   3   5   7   9   10   8   6   4   2

A portion of this book first appeared in *Family Circle*.

Grateful acknowledgment is made for permission to use the following copyrighted works:
Selections from *Guided Meditations, Explorations and Healings* by Stephen Levine. Copyright © 1991 by Stephen Levine. Used by permission of Doubleday, a division of Random House, Inc.
Selections from *Rituals of Healing* by Jeanne Achterberg, Barbara Dossey, and Leslie Kolkmeier. Copyright © 1994 by Jeanne Achterberg, Barbara Dossey, and Leslie Kolkmeier. Used by permission of Bantam Books, a division of Random House, Inc.
Selections from *The Dance of Anger* by Harriet Goldhor Lerner. Copyright © 1985 by Harriet G. Lerner. Reprinted by permission of HarperCollins Publishers, Inc.
Adaptation of selections from *52 Silly Things to Do When You Are Blue* by Lynn Gordon. Copyright © 1994 by Lynn Gordon. Used by permission of Chronicle Books, San Francisco.

LIBRARY OF CONGRESS CATALOGING-IN-PUBLICATION DATA
Domar, Alice D.
Self-nurture : learning to care for youself as effectively as
you care for everyone else / Alice D. Domar and Henry Dreher.
p.   cm.
ISBN 0-670-88286-0
1. Women—Psychology.   2. Women—Conduct of life.   3. Nurturing behavior.
4. Self-help techniques.   I. Dreher, Henry.   II. Title.
HQ1206.D64   2000
305.42—dc21   99–16823

This book is printed on acid-free paper.

Printed in the United States of America
Set in Minion • Designed by Francesca Belanger

To Mom and Ricky, and in memory of Dad
—A.D.D.

For my sister, Stephanie Krotick
—H.D.

Authors' Note

THE NAMES and identifying details of the patients and some friends discussed in the book have been changed to protect anonymity. The sections in this book on mind-body medical techniques are offered as health recommendations, not as substitutes for conventional medical therapies for disease. We recommend that you utilize these approaches only in conjunction with—not instead of—mainstream medicine. Consult your physician about any symptom or illness you may have and inform him or her about any treatments you embark on.

Acknowledgments

I WOULD LIKE TO THANK all of the women who have taught me so much about the power of self-care. These include my patients, who allowed me to try to help them learn to care for themselves, and women who came to hear me speak at conferences and workshops and guided me, through their questions and reactions to what I was saying, to speak more forcefully about not feeling guilty about meeting one's own needs.

The women who comprise the team at the Mind/Body Center for Women's Health are an inspiration. Their dedication and passion to improve the physical and psychological health of women is visible not only through hard work but also through their humor and compassion. I could not have created this book without the ideas and input of Patty Martin Arcari, R.N., Ph.D., Michele Chausse, Jan Cook, M.D., Lisa Conboy, M.A., Brenda Coyle, Ph.D, Karen Fasciano, Ph.D, Melissa Freizinger, M.A., Leslee Kagan, R.N., M.S., N.P., Amora Magna, Maureen McCormick, Ph.D, Jana Morra, Ph.D, the Reverend Barbara Nielsen, Eileen O'Connell, R.N., M.S.N., Sara Orozco, Ph.D, Harriet Redmond, M.S., R.N., C.S., Eva Selhub, M.D., Ellen Slawsby, Ph.D, Edee Simon-Israel, M.B.A., Heather Von Bergen, Ann Webster, Ph.D, and Tricia Zuttermeister, M.A.

I would also like to thank Herbert Benson, M.D., and Marilyn Wilcher for their support, friendship, and trust.

My husband, David Ostrow, and daughter, Sarah Domar Ostrow, deserve major kudos for their patience and tolerance of the time it took away from them for me to complete this book. Their love, understanding, and hugs were more than appreciated.

And finally, I would like to acknowledge the enthusiastic support of all of my friends and specific ideas from several of them: Betsy Anderson, Nancy Denardo, Carolyn Horn, Betsy Loring Matyas, Karen Sothern, Linda Tischler, and Karen Whitney.

—Alice D. Domar, Ph.D.

I WISH TO THANK Dr. Domar's patients and the women who have been kind and courageous enough to openly share their experiences with me. I am grateful to several people who gave me various kinds of nurturing support as I worked on this project, including Barbara Miller, Harris Dienstfrey, Nurit Koppel, and Bruce McCarty. I owe a debt of thanks to three individuals, leaders in the mind-body field who have helped me understand what it means to self-nurture and who have been ceaseless sources of inspiration to me as a writer and thinker: Lydia Temoshok, James Pennebaker, and George F. Solomon. My gratitude to Therese Brown, for her marvelous work as tape transcriber. Finally, my deepest thanks and love to my wife, Deborah Chiel, who has nurtured me and this project in countless ways.

—Henry Dreher

WE WOULD BOTH LIKE TO THANK the women who shared their stories for this book. This includes a number of Ali's patients as well as her mother and sister. We know that it can be very difficult to be interviewed about personal issues, knowing that each story will be read by many other women.

Our agents, Chris Tomasino and Jonathan Diamond, were, as always, enthusiastic, supportive, critical when we needed it, and good friends throughout. Their comments and intuition were invaluable.

Our editor Pam Dorman has been exceptional. Her ability to take a manuscript, which we thought was just fine, and tweak and alter here and there to make it even better, was incredible. We would also like to thank others at Viking Penguin, including Susan

Hans O'Connor and Mindy Werner as well as all of the rest of the team who supported us along the way.

And finally, to our spouses, David Ostrow and Deborah Chiel, for their editing, proofreading, and rewriting suggestions, as well as their love.

—*Alice D. Domar, Ph.D., and Henry Dreher*

Contents

1

INTRODUCTION:

WHY SELF-NURTURE?

❦ ❦

HAVE YOU EVER EXPERIENCED one of those moments when after thinking and thinking about a problem for days and days, maybe even dreaming about it, then suddenly something triggers this amazing insight and you either solve the problem or at least understand why you were so bothered by it?

Well, this happened to me recently. The event that triggered the sudden insight was my mother's purchase of a swing set for my daughter Sarah's second birthday. Sarah is crazy for swings, and she was ecstatic to have a swingset in her own backyard. She begged to go outside, and once happily perched on a swing, demanded constant pushing. As I pushed her (and pushed her, and pushed her), I had a sudden flashback to my childhood in Concord, Massachusetts.

We lived in a rural area and the family next door had five children, the youngest of whom, Ann, was a year older than I. Ann was my best friend. Her father built this amazing swing in the woods behind their house. The swing was supported by very long ropes, suspended from a towering tree, high on a hill. When you were pushed on that swing, you really felt as if you were flying.

But we weren't old enough to have truly mastered the art of pumping, so we needed one of Ann's older brothers to push us in order to reach breathtaking heights.

Ann and I would beg her brothers incessantly to push us. Day in and day out we would hunt them down in the house and, without any inhibition, plead with them to come out to the swing and push.

This is the sudden insight that I had while pushing Sarah. Looking back, what I find utterly remarkable was our total lack of hesitation about beseeching Ann's brothers to do something for us that was strictly for our own enjoyment. What boldness! But could I ever imagine myself doing the same thing now? Of course not. I would feel selfish.

This got me thinking about the course of female development from childhood through adolescence to young adulthood. Why do we lose the sense that we are entitled to joy for its own sake? What happens to our willingness to ask others to help meet our needs? When do we start to feel guilty about pursuing pleasure and play? At what stage of development do we adopt the belief that our larger purpose is to serve everyone else's needs?

The answers can be found by questioning our roles as self-sacrificing caretakers, family stabilizers in a world that still views men as the primary breadwinners. Experts on women's development have explored these issues in depth. That's not my purpose with this book. My purpose is to empower women to overcome this cultural legacy. The memory of my own early ability to seek joy as a child intensifies my desire to help women nurture themselves and ask others for nurturance.

In our development as women, obviously we must shed many of our childlike attributes. But we must also hold fast to some of them. The most fully-realized women hold on to their childhood pluck and spontaneity. These are women, I have found, who can nurture themselves—women who might take an hour to read a book without feeling guilty, or call up a group of friends on a whim and convince them to go out and do something. These women retain their childhood spark.

I am reminded again of my memory of Ann's brothers and the swing. My goal for myself, my patients, and my readers is that we manage to hang onto that pure joy, that ability to take flight. We may stop swinging but we don't have to stop soaring—in our creative imaginations, careers, sex lives, relationships, or spiritual endeavors. To take flight, though, we must develop what psychotherapist Lawrence LeShan calls a "fierce and tender concern" for every facet of *our* being. That fierce and tender concern is what I call *self-nurture*.

WHAT DO WOMEN NEED?

Sigmund Freud's famous question, "What do women want?" is something I've wondered about myself. During my thirteen years as a health psychologist specializing in women's well-being, I have settled on a slightly different question: "What do women really need?" What women *need* is to learn how to nurture themselves. We need to shower as much loving kindness on ourselves as we habitually shower on loved ones, and even not-so-loved ones. We need to be loved for our fully formed selves, not for our dependent, appeasing selves. And the only way we can have fully formed selves is by granting ourselves the same tenderness and fierce protectiveness we'd otherwise reserve for a beloved child.

I have discovered these seemingly simple truths in my own life, and I have rediscovered them thousands of times in my work with patients. I am considered an expert in stress management for women, and I have come to realize that all the relaxation techniques in the world won't amount to any true relaxation if they are not guided by self-nurturance. When self-nurture is the underlying principle behind stress management, the healing effect of mind-body techniques—from relaxation to cognitive restructuring to prayer—is exponentially enhanced. Hence, *Self-Nurture* is a hands-on guide to creative, emotional, and spiritual self-care.

I've designed the book to help you cultivate self-nurture over the course of one year, with two different theme areas (chapters) for each of the four seasons.

- Winter begins with an introduction to mind-body nurture, including basic techniques you can apply throughout the book. The second "winter" chapter focuses on your role as a mother and/or daughter, showing how you can nurture self within the family unit.
- Spring is the season of renewal, so I start with a chapter on the sacred body, in which you learn to shift from bodily shame to celebration. To renew relationships, and nurture existing ones, turn to the next chapter on love mates (self-nurture with or without significant others).
- Summer represents free time for the soul; it includes chapters on creativity and leisure ("child's play") and friendships and sibling relationships ("the social safety net").
- Autumn, often a period of new beginnings, includes a chapter to help you safeguard your soul on the job ("joy at work") and a final chapter on how to develop a self-nurturing spirituality.

Each chapter is filled with exercises and explorations that help you to become more self-nurturing in that particular area. If you spend about six weeks implementing the suggestions in each of the next eight chapters, the entire program of self-nurture will last a year.

I offer this seasonal structure because it places the primary themes of women's lives in an order and context that makes sense for many of us. But don't feel obliged to follow this structure. Rather, I suggest that you identify the areas of your life where you most require self-nurturance, and concentrate on those first. For instance, if you have serious trouble with body-nurture but are very self-nurturing in the context of your marriage, you may wish to spend two months on the body chapter and no time on the "love mates" chapter.

So take a month or two to work on each of these issues, skipping any areas that are not relevant to you, while spending additional weeks or months on facets of your life that call out for care and attention. As you shift your focus to different realms of your life (i.e., from the body to spirituality to creativity), try to sustain transformations you've made from previous realms. Imagine that you are adding layers of positive change to your life; that is how self-nurture can become a natural, on-going process. Once you commit to self-nurture, you become empowered to solve stubborn problems and relieve your own suffering.

I have seen it time and again: women who live with passive, self-negating thoughts such as "Who will love me?" "Who will solve my problems?" Whether they suffer from job burnout, marital discord, loneliness, infertility, financial pressures, boredom, flagging self-esteem, chronic pain, or illness, problems are resolved and pain is relieved once they commit themselves to self-nurture. Our work together empowers them to shift from this external orientation to an internal one: "How can I nurture myself?" It's a profoundly healing transformation. This book is a hands-on guide enabling you to make this shift in every facet of your life.

For the past decade, I have led the women's health programs at the Beth Israel Deaconess Medical Center's Division of Behavioral Medicine at Harvard Medical School. I have directed research and group programs for women dealing with infertility, menopause, and PMS. On a group or individual basis, I have treated women with every type of women's health problem. I currently head Harvard's newly formed

Mind-Body Center for Women's Health, at the Mind-Body Medical Institute, a unique effort to study and provide mind-body medicine to
women.

What is mind-body medicine? Any method in which the mind is
mobilized in the treatment of a physical disorder. The most common
mind-body techniques are relaxation (including varieties of meditation,
imagery, yoga, and deep breathing); cognitive therapy (transforming
negative thought patterns); emotional expression; skills for communication and coping; and spiritual practices, including prayer. Although I
teach all these methods, I now believe that self-nurture is the overriding
principle that must bind together any successful program of mind-body
medicine, whether for women recovering from illness or healthy women
who want to live the healthiest, most joyful lives.

I have been asked why I am so committed to self-nurture. Part of my
philosophy grows out of my family life. The other is a direct response to
the enthusiasm of my patients and other women for this approach.
Three years ago, when I began to speak about self-nurture, the number of women who showed up for my lectures surprised me, as did the
passionate intensity of their reactions. It didn't matter whether they
were professionals, medical patients, or members of the public. Invariably, people rushed up to me afterward to say that they felt I was talking
personally to them—about their lives, relationships, and most fervent
desires.

When I talk about self-nurturance, I don't mean just buying yourself material things or learning how to spend money on yourself. I speak
to women from all walks of life, from the inner city to the most comfortable of suburbs. The basic philosophy is to learn how to care for yourself.
At a recent workshop for African American women at a neighborhood
health clinic, the participants told of a lifetime of caring for others. Several women spoke of simultaneously caring for elderly parents, children,
and grandchildren. The classic image of freedom "when the children are
grown" doesn't hold for them. Yet we successfully brainstormed ways
they could better care for themselves, ranging from spending more time
for prayers to learning when to leave an unsatisfactory relationship.
The philosophy of self-nurture spoke to these women, as it does to all
women, regardless of income, race, or background.

WHY I TEACH SELF-NURTURE

I remember clearly the moment when I recognized self-nurture as the essence of effective stress management for women. It occurred in 1987, my first year as a clinician in the Division of Behavioral Medicine at Beth Israel Deaconess Medical Center, when I first led a mind-body group for women with infertility. In the years since, one of my specialties has been treating women with infertility, an extreme model for the stresses women experience in everyday life. These women often feel out of control, demoralized, burned out, maritally challenged, and angry over the loss of their childbearing capacity. At the beginning, however, it took me a while to grasp the issues at stake for these women.

I was coleader of that first group in 1987, playing second fiddle to my colleague, Steve Maurer, since at the time I had little experience running groups by myself. My purpose as a facilitator was to provide the female perspective for a group of women experiencing a uniquely female form of suffering. But Steve took the lead in teaching mind-body techniques, such as relaxation, coping skills, and cognitive restructuring. Less than an hour before the fourth group session, I received a call from Steve.

"I have the flu, and I'm much too sick to come in tonight," he said.

It was too late to call the patients and cancel. "I can't do this, Steve," I said nervously. I had never taught cognitive restructuring, and though I understood the concepts, I wasn't prepared to conduct the session.

I clearly recall Steve's advice. "Just think of something you feel you can teach and do that." He hung up, and I scanned my mind for anything that would help this group of women who felt so miserable and out of control. It was one of those moments when desperation forces you to look within yourself and ask fundamental questions. I asked myself, "What can I offer the group members that they won't get in the rest of this program?" and "What do they really need most?"

The first thought that popped into my head was that these women, whose suffering I had come to understand during the first few sessions, did not know how to nurture themselves. Yes, we were teaching them methods for mental and physical relaxation, techniques to combat negative thinking. But we had not acknowledged that guilt, low self-esteem, and other legacies from their personal histories seemed to disable them from taking good care of themselves. They did not know how to say no to family, friends, and spouses, nor did they carve out nearly enough time for relaxation and pleasure. In many cases, their shaky self-esteems were built on rickety foundations: feeling worthwhile only as caretakers, whether at home or at work, with even the tiniest lapse spurring anxiety or depression. If in their own eyes they fell short as wives, daughters, sisters, coworkers, or friends, they did not deserve anything substantial for themselves. An inability to bear children was only one more example of their shortcomings.

With these thoughts came clarity about my mission. I began that evening's group by suggesting to the participants that we focus on how they could take better care of themselves. This simple comment sparked a lively discussion. The women began to confront how difficult it was for them to self-nurture, how little time they took for themselves, how guilty they felt engaging in activities solely for their own enjoyment. The collective outpouring was both cathartic and therapeutic. But I did not want us to get stuck at the level of problem-naming. I wanted to move them toward problem-solving. So I suggested that we brainstorm for practical ways they could care for themselves without excessive guilt.

While the women eventually had fun doing this, at first they were taken aback by the whole discussion. But as they talked, they embraced self-nurture as if it were a missing piece in their struggle to cope with the stress and sadness associated with their fertility struggles. Many of the women were willing to contemplate this thought: If I can bestow tenderness on myself, maybe I can get through this terrible trial. Maybe I can get through just about anything.

Most of the ideas were stunningly simple. Here are a few examples:
- Take myself to a movie that I want to see.
- Buy myself a bouquet of flowers after a rough day at work.
- Make time every night for a hot bath with mineral salts, by candlelight.
- Eat a bowl of ice cream once in a while without punishing myself with harsh tirades about fat, heart disease, and cancer.
- Buy myself a hammock so I can lounge away Sunday afternoons.
- Take an evening every week for yoga, qi gong, or t'ai chi classes.
- Get a full body massage every two weeks instead of once a year.
- Read the novel that has been sitting by my bedside for ten months.

Most of us can identify with the desire to nurture ourselves in these ways, and I encourage you to make your own lists. But these women discovered that the specific forms of self-soothing were less important than making a broader transformation in their daily lives.

By the end of the session, the women pledged to follow through on their self-nurturing proposals. But their promises did not come easily. They were hesitant for several reasons about whether they'd be able to stick to their plans. They weren't sure they could remain sufficiently guilt-free to enjoy their self-nurturing activities. They weren't sure they could find enough time. They weren't sure their families would accept them taking "extra" time for themselves. Their responses presaged the fearful concerns I would hear from women whenever I have taught self-nurture in the decade since. That's when I realized that self-nurture could not be viewed as just another technique. It would require lifelong commitment, much the way a healthy diet requires lifelong commitment, lest we succumb to a sense of helplessness after the failure of yet another faddish quick fix.

Despite these concerns, on their part and mine, something exciting had happened that evening. I'd managed, through a mixture of desperation and intuition, to touch a deep chord in this group of women. In turn, they had responded with self-awareness and a willingness to change their habitual patterns. I believed I had hit upon the missing link in our program. What I experienced and learned that first night changed my approach to almost all of my patients, so that now self-nurture underlies my entire practice of mind-body medicine.

My Own Journey to Self-Nurture

In looking back at my family life, I've come to see the origins of both my difficulties and successes with self-care. Like an artist who later in life comes to understand the hidden meanings in an early work, I have glimpsed some insights as to why self-nurture was the first idea that popped into my head running that group in 1987, and why I have pursued this thread ever since.

My parents were married for fifty-one years until my father's death several years ago. My father, born in Russia, was a leading economist and teacher at M.I.T. who made important contributions to economic theory. He was a loving though strict father, and like many fathers of the 1950s, he was hardly involved in child-rearing. I always recall my mother saying that he never once changed a diaper. My mother and her family, who came to this country from Germany during the war, had barely escaped the concentration camps. (My grandfather managed to get out of a concentration camp in France, and the members of my mother's family reunited in Richmond, Virginia.) My mother's experiences in Nazi Germany sharpened her survival instincts. "We'd go to the movies or swimming and there would be a sign, 'No Jews Allowed,' " she told me. "That kind of thing hit you almost every day. It either makes you or breaks you."

My mother's toughness served her well in this country. Both my parents were devoted to my older sister and me, but it was my mother who shouldered the major responsibility for raising us. By the time I started first grade, my mother did something no other mothers I knew had tried—she went to graduate school, and eventually received her master's degree in social work. By the time I was ten, she was working full-time and returning home with a slim fifteen minutes to spare before 5:45— the appointed dinner time my father insisted upon.

I had a naive preteen impression that my mother cut corners as a housewife: she was always the first on the block to embrace those time-saving innovations of the sixties and seventies—the Veg-o-Matics and Hamburger Helpers. When I was a teenager, I recall our family getting a microwave—a space-age device I'd never seen in anyone else's house. I now realize that my mother was simply making do—having a career, which to her meant a chance for a creative and independent life, and taking care of her family, which meant getting dinner on the table by 5:45.

As I grew up, my mother took increasing steps toward independence. Triple-duty as a wife, mother, and social worker was both pleasurable and burdensome. Today she insists that she didn't mind all that juggling because she so loved and enjoyed her husband and kids, and I certainly believe her. But she did mind some of my father's rigidity, and by the time I was a teenager she insisted on more freedom to pursue her own interests and desires. My parents' unspoken bargain was clear: For continuing to shoulder all of the home-related responsibilities, my mother would get a great deal more autonomy in her everyday activities.

I remember a turning point in my parents' relationship—and my mother's development. It was my senior year in high school, and several friends and I had saved enough money to take a weeklong trip to Bermuda. My mother wanted to join us for the first few days, and I was delighted. But my father wasn't. It wasn't that he wanted to join us; he just didn't want my mother going without him. I recall them fighting for days over this issue. Eventually, my mother won. She flew with my friends and me to Bermuda and we had a blast.

For some time afterward, my parents skirmished over similar issues. One battle involved our family's usual mountain-hiking vacations. After my mother was injured in a car accident, she could no longer hike. Yet we'd still take these trips, and my mother would remain in our cabin while the rest of us spent the day trekking. My mother tells me that things changed when she decided not to *ask* for a different arrangement but rather to *demand* one. "I told my husband, 'I'm going to rent a cottage on Cape Cod for the kids and me, and you're welcome to come.' I did not say 'May I?' I said this is what we are going to do. Of course, he eventually decided to come along. But this time I made the decision."

My father, a product of his time and culture, was never going to become a nineties man, doing some housework and child-rearing. But my mother wanted him to accept her freedom to have a rich life. She eventually won this struggle, and in later years my mother never looked back. She sometimes took vacations without my father, did extensive volunteer work, and had a successful career as a social worker and therapist that filled her days with meaningful work. My mother offers this succinct summary of her marriage to my father: "You know, he loved me very much. But I was resolute, and it opened his eyes. He realized that I had my needs, and it was time that I did what I really wanted to do."

Looking back, I realize how strongly I identified with my mother's struggle, and how it shaped my later work and philosophy. In my preschool years, I had the example of a loving mother who sacrificed everything for her family. As a school-age child, I had the example of a mother who, like so many mothers today, juggled career and family, taking on multiple duties with boundless energy and aplomb. As I got older, though, I recognized the toll it took on her. I was upset with my father for his inflexibility, and I empathized with my mother's predicament. My mother was in a marriage with a man she loved and who tried to meet her needs as best he could. It just wasn't enough. After a rocky period of transformation, however, my parents' marriage became more stable, not less.

I can look back and recognize now that my mother's struggle was highly specific, and in its specificity I learned the lesson of self-nurture. Namely, she had never demanded that my father fulfill her needs with more love, support, provisions, or quality time. She already had these. She wanted him to recognize her right to pursue sources of joy both inside and outside the marriage. She didn't need his permission, but she did need his acceptance, lest the marriage crumble. My mother's "triumph" not only strengthened my parents' marriage; it made them both better people.

Having witnessed my mother's gradual transformation, I internalized the message that women have a right to meet their own needs. Moreover, under the right circumstances and with the right intent, staking this claim strengthens rather than destroys relationships. As a teenager, I recognized my mother's increasing happiness and well-being, and I knew it was because she had "won" the freedom to cultivate sources of pleasure and meaning that did not depend on my father.

I learned self-nurture from my mother in other ways that I probably absorbed without realizing it. She reminds me that as a teenager, I was one of several local kids who babysat for a group of mentally handicapped preschoolers. Why was I given this job? My mother was running a support group for the mothers of these children, and every six weeks she took them on day-long excursions to museums, to the country, on ski trips. It was my mother's idea to give these women opportunities to take time out from their caretaking responsibilities, to leave behind their daily chores in order to simply enjoy themselves. What did this accomplish? In my mother's words, "It opened their eyes to the fact that they could still have lives of their own."

My mother still meets with five of the women from her original group. Twenty-four years later, they retain a bond of understanding and a commitment to good times together. Clearly, she's been teaching self-nurture in her own inimitable way.

My mother did not become self-nurturing by cutting herself off from my father. On the contrary, she met her needs both apart from and together with him. You will learn throughout this book that self-care has two aspects: one in solitude, one in relationship. The mere phrase "self-nurture" may conjure images of time alone—taking hot baths, meditating, renting movies. But self-nurture doesn't just mean private time to tend to one's needs. Self-nurture also means taking care of ourselves in our relationships with significant others, family members, friends. Too often, our relationships are characterized by the rituals of obligation— we only spend time with relatives on holidays, with spouses at supper, with friends at dinner parties. It is the height of self-nurture to carve out time with loved ones solely to confide, "catch up," or enjoy an artistic or utterly frivolous event with each other.

"All persons need both relationships and solitude," says psychotherapist Lawrence LeShan. "The question is how to find the right balance." Each chapter in this book, devoted to a different realm of women's lives, will help you cultivate self-nurture both in solitude and with others. For instance, developing self-nurture at work often means two things. First, we can take time for ourselves, away from the workday craziness, to take a mindful walk around the block. But we can also take time with a colleague to go to lunch, schmooze, laugh, and relax together away from the workplace.

Self-nurture is not about being selfish. It is about self-care.

WHY CAN'T ALL WOMEN SELF-NURTURE?

Why do some women have so much trouble with self-nurture? The answer can only be found in each of our personal histories. Nevertheless, our families and our culture have (sometimes unwittingly) conditioned women to be self-denying, caretaking, appeasing, and people-pleasing. The simple but devastating message we're brought up to believe is that if we nurture ourselves we are being selfish.

I have bought into this fiction myself, and it has taken years of committed introspection for me to mostly overcome it. Even so, I still sometimes struggle with guilt when I take time to nurture myself. A year ago, I had surgery to remove my gall bladder. After returning home from the hospital, I had a week off from work to recover. My surgeon specifically told me not to try to do too much, to give my body as much rest and relaxation as possible. I cannot remember a time when I felt so guilt-free about doing nothing. "Doctor's orders!" I thought. Someone I respected, a person with authority, had commanded me to kick back for a week. During the first few days I felt too draggy to leave bed, so I watched TV and read. Later I spent time reading on our porch. Beyond that, I didn't do much. And I enjoyed every minute of the nothingness. Without the surgeon's prescription, I'd never have been able to goof off, without guilt, for even one day. When I'm well, and have no "excuse," I still have to convince myself that an hour stolen for pure self-nurture is not selfish, that it is good for me, and hence, good for those around me, as well.

The fact that I know better—that I'm an expert in women's stress and an advocate of self-nurture—doesn't mean I've been able to cleanse myself of the personal and social taboos against women taking time solely for their own well-being.

Too many of my patients and friends struggle with the same impediments. Why should we have to be seriously ill before we give ourselves full permission to unwind? Why should we brand ourselves selfish whenever we seek pleasure that has nothing to do with giving, producing, or caretaking? We should not. And yet, regardless of the nature of their problem—from garden-variety stress to life-threatening disease—I meet the same resistances in women when I first talk about self-nurture:

> "How can I take time for X when my baby needs me? It would be so selfish."
>
> "How can I go off and do X when my husband gets so little quality time with me? It would be so self-obsessed."
>
> "How can I tell my mother that I can't do X for her because I want to do X for myself? It would be so uncaring."
>
> "It would be disgusting of me to ever indulge my desire for X food. How could I be such a pig?"
>
> "I can't ask for X during sex. It would be too self-centered."
>
> "Who am I to take vacation when I'm so strapped for cash? How self-indulgent."
>
> "Who am I not to help my sibling when he/she so desperately needs me? It would be so narcissistic."

These judgments usually sound to us like voices of reason, sharp but sensible echoes of common sense and moral correctness. In truth, they are harsh rebukes of any rising impulse to treat ourselves with tenderness. I hope this book will help you discover the origins of your self-negating voices, teaching you not only how to label them but how to silence them for good.

After a recent self-nurture workshop, a tall, striking forty-something woman from Texas stood up and asked me a wise question. "How can I make sure that my fifteen-year-old daughter has more self-esteem than I do?" My answer was simple: Be the right kind of role model. If your daughter sees you taking good care of yourself, it will teach her the meaning of self-regard. As long as you are essentially available, she won't feel robbed when you take time for yourself. Rather, you'll have provided her with a worthy example to emulate. Also, carving out time for your own relaxation, pleasure, and creativity will enhance the quality of your time with your daughter, because you'll be stronger and more present when you are with her. Selfless, self-denying mothers are exhausted and resentful. Self-nurturing mothers are energetic, aware, and open-hearted.

DEFINING GENUINE SELF-NURTURE

You may think, "But I know women who constantly nurture themselves, and they still seem stressed out." You may even see yourself as one of these women. Often, however, when I get to know such women I discover that their brand of self-nurture is anything but nourishing.

Some women "nurture" themselves with material goods—new clothes, shoes, furnishings, artwork, fabulous trips, and entertainment. But compulsive quests for material possessions often betray a lack rather than an abundance of self-esteem. Frequently, these women feel empty inside, and their attempts to fill that emptiness can't succeed because the void is emotional or spiritual rather than material. On the other hand, many women with less money feel guilty spending *anything* on themselves. For them, shopping for modestly priced items strictly for their own pleasure can be a liberating experience.

Other patients and women I've known appear to be anything but self-negating; their surface behavior is narcissistic. But those of us who grasp ceaselessly for ourselves never feel satisfied because we're still looking outside for nurturance. And we're chronically ticked off when that nurturance isn't forthcoming or doesn't gratify us. Here again, what passes for self-nurture is actually self-destructive. Of course we need nurturance from others, but people with narcissistic needs have old wounds that have not healed. Material goods and other people's attention temporarily salve the old wounds but never truly heal them.

Elaine, a forty-six-year-old patient, had an out-of-control shopping habit. But she was not rich, and the credit cards and department store bills began to accumulate. Eventually, she took an extra job—one she profoundly disliked—just to pay these bills! After working with me, Elaine came to realize that chronic unhappiness in her marriage, and her own inability to nurture on both emotional and spiritual levels, was the underlying cause of her addictive shopping. The only way to heal old wounds that cause us to grasp for love or possessions is to recognize them, grieve for our losses, and nourish ourselves with compassion.

When I speak about self-nurture, some ask, "What about helping others?" I strongly believe that our highest instincts for helping—reaching out to loved ones and strangers—are fed rather than hindered by self-nurture. I'm not the first to notice this seeming paradox, but I've seen it play itself out clearly in my patients' lives. When caught up in the caretaking syndrome, they are beset by fatigue, boredom, and resentment. Their ceaseless giving, predominantly motivated by guilt and obligation, ultimately disables them from giving *well.* Once they start focusing on their needs, and meet them assertively and tenderly, then their whole orientation shifts, and their giving impulses become grounded in self-esteem and openheartedness. They no longer feel, consciously or unconsciously, that they're being ripped off or sucked dry. These women discover that genuine self-nurture is the polar opposite of narcissism; it lays the ground for an altruism of the heart.

MEETING OUR NEEDS IN THE NEW MILLENNIUM

Two generations ago, American women (and men, for that matter) grew up in stronger, more supportive social networks. The web of interconnections was broader, and our communities were comprised of tightly knit extended families. Despite their often constricted roles and marriages, our mothers and grandmothers had their emotional and spiritual needs met by many more women—their sisters and aunts and female cousins and grandmothers who either lived with them or in their neighborhoods. These women cared for each other in crises, and on a daily basis. They took care of each others' babies, cooked meals for each other, and shared each others' joys and sorrows. By the 1970s, the fabric of family unity and support began to fray, and with that sociological development came a new wrinkle on the old man-woman story.

Before, women were wholly dependent on men to meet their economic needs, but primary emotional needs were often gratified by the nearby community of women. In the past three decades, massive social changes have enabled women to become more economically independent, but the breakup of traditional extended families and neighborhoods has made it harder for women to have their emotional needs met by other women. We began to think that the men in our lives should meet all our needs.

It's taken women several decades to recognize that no man, no matter how strong or sensitive, can meet all our needs. So women of the new millennium find themselves stuck in a bind: we no longer have the same strong-knit communities of women, nor do we have the illusion of perfect multifaceted men who can take care of us financially and emotionally. Who, then, is going to satisfy our many needs and desires? The best answer I can offer is an old Wall Street pointer: diversify, diversify. We should recognize that different needs will be met by different people, including our partners, family members, friends—and ourselves. This realization is liberating in an era when it's too much to expect any one person or institution to fulfill every part of our complex selves.

Many of my patients have yet to discover these truths, and this causes much suffering. They say, "My husband [or mother/father/friend/lover] doesn't understand me. He is just not meeting my needs." More and more, I find myself responding, "Maybe he just can't meet those needs. Maybe he just doesn't know how." I counsel them to accept the person's limits, then turn to others and themselves to meet those needs. When they make this shift, they often report the same experience: a growing sense of inner freedom. If the relationship has redeeming value, it will more likely survive, and often thrive, no longer carrying an excessive and unrealistic burden.

Nonetheless, I've certainly had patients whose transformations caused strain in their relationships, particularly with spouses or partners. Throughout this book, and particularly in chapter 5, "Love Mates: Self-Nurture with (or Without) Significant Others," I will discuss how women can prevent their efforts at self-nurture from causing severe imbalances in their marriages and partnerships. Some men are threatened by changes in their partners, who not only spend more time on themselves but begin to assert their needs more forcefully. These men are not usually disturbed by the extra time a woman takes for a hot bath, meditation, or lunch with friends. They're really bothered by her heightened self-esteem, since it alters the dynamics of the relationship. While friction often accompanies positive change, there are ways for women to guard against disruptive conflict with significant others. Communication skills are key, but the best way to guard against serious trouble with loved ones is to take them with you on your transformative journey. I'll describe how you can accomplish this end.

SURVIVING AS A JUGGLER

Imagine for a moment that you had been invited to meet with the president and top White House officials. What would be the first issue you'd want to discuss with them? A recent U.S. government survey asked this question of 250,000 working women, and the number-one topic they mentioned was their inability to balance work and family. The respondents also said that stress was the most pressing problem they faced in their everyday lives.

We're all familiar with the proverbial juggling act. As a working mother who juggles many roles, I am well aware of the dizzying stresses caused by conditions we face today. I recently heard a very scary statistic that illustrates the magnitude of the strain women are feeling. An NBC News report cited the fact that since 1975, the rate of women dying in automobile accidents has skyrocketed. In the past two decades, the mortality rate for men in car accidents has declined 10 percent, while it has increased 66 percent for women! The statisticians discovered that more women drivers on the road was not the overriding factor in this tragic rise. The investigators could come up with only one theory: Women were so stressed out from increasing social pressures and multiple roles that it was causing them to drive too fast and too recklessly! You can imagine that my jaw dropped, but not in disbelief. This alarming statistic only confirmed what I already believed to be true.

Much has changed between men and women. Yet women still shoulder the lion's share of responsibility for both child care and housework. Research in the early 1990s revealed that new mothers spend nearly four times as many hours per day in infant care than fathers. Moreover, many new mothers must still work—if not immediately then soon after their newborns' arrivals. "Although two out of three mothers work outside the home, it seems that many of them are trying to do more for their children, not less," wrote social psychologist Carin Rubenstein in a 1998 column in *The New York Times*. Since women are spending more time at work and with children, our crowded schedules can become unbearably tight. It's no wonder that we feel perennially exhausted and unappreciated.

Finding time to breathe, let alone think, is a first-order concern when we lead such hectic lives. Even before the birth of my daughter, I rarely felt I had enough time for my husband, friends, family, and creative pursuits. In addition to being a wife and mother, I am a sister, a friend, and a daughter. Last but not least, I am a professional woman whose work entails not only group and individual sessions with patients, but teaching, research, administrative tasks, lectures, meetings, travel, and media appearances.

In my life, a good example of non-self-nurturing priorities was my behavior during my own honeymoon in Greece. I will always recall the look on my husband's face when he ambled back into our hotel room and found me busily writing lists of things to do when we got home. "What's on that list?" he asked. "Oh, buying pillows to match the new sofa, writing thank-you notes for our wedding gifts, that sort of thing." He couldn't believe that I was taking time away from enjoying our honeymoon to worry about pillows, thank-you notes, and other remarkably trivial items. In retrospect, I can't believe it either. (Incidentally, it took five years before I found the time to search for just the right pillows.)

It's as though our nervous systems have been hard-wired to fret over mental lists—to remain vigilant lest we forget to meet a deadline, pay a bill, pick up a child. So vigilant, in fact, that we are capable of losing ourselves in anxious preoccupation, until we find ourselves making lists on our honeymoons. But we can rewire our systems by restoring contact with parts of ourselves that can fully breathe, think, relax, and self-nurture.

We can also learn better ways of coping with the inevitable stresses associated with juggling. We can develop what I call discoverable strengths. These strengths enable us to change our relationship to people and events, so we not only seem to have more control over the swirl of events in our daily dramas, we actually exercise more control. Without these strengths, even minor stresses—such as a boss's criticism, a husband's irritability, a child's dropped glass—can cause us to become unraveled.

The discoverable strengths include planning, setting priorities, problem-solving, support-seeking, self-soothing, calm reflectiveness, independent thinking, moral conviction, emotional expression, tact, honesty, fighting spirit, and spiritual intelligence. How do we discover these strengths in ourselves? Self-nurture is the final pathway, because it grants us the time and space to make the inward journey.

With a daily ritual of self-care, an inner worthiness begins to blossom. Once it does, you'll make the right decisions on your own behalf. You will find the courage to act in ways that are self-expressive and self-protective. You will start caring for each part of yourself with a fierce and tender concern.

The Corners of the Soul

The stress that arises from participation in multiple roles leads some women to wish they could pull back from work or family obligations. But pulling back is rarely a solution. Margaret Mietus Sanik, Associate Professor of Family Resource Management at Cornell University, has uncovered evidence that full-time homemakers experience higher levels of psychological distress than working women who also have families. Apparently, multiple roles may be stressful, but they can also lead to richer, more satisfying lives.

Remarkable evidence for the life-affirming, health-enhancing benefits of multiple roles was published in 1998 in the prestigious *Journal of the American Medical Association.* Leading mind-body scientist Sheldon Cohen of Carnegie Mellon University gave 276 healthy volunteers nasal drops containing cold viruses, followed them to see who developed colds, and then measured their severity. Before this experiment, Cohen asked the volunteers to report on their sources of social support. His hypothesis was that people with more support would have stronger immune systems and, hence, greater resistance to colds. After analyzing his data, he found that certain individuals did resist colds, but they were not those who simply had more people in their support networks. Rather, they had more diverse networks—they turned to many different sources of support, such as spouses, parents, friends, workmates, and other members of their social group. Specifically, people with only one to three types of social ties were four times more likely to catch a serious cold than people with six or more types of ties.

Cohen's hardy volunteers engaged in multiple roles, exercising different aspects of their personalities in a range of relationships. Patricia Linville, Ph.D., uses the lovely term "self-complexity" to describe people who live out their multifaceted identities. Dr. Linville has also shown that such "complex" people are psychologically and physically healthier than their less complex counterparts. But here's a paradox: Self-complexity serves us well if we keep it simple—not trying to do more than we can, just doing as much as we can to remain curious, excited, challenged, and alive.

To live out these roles, we may wish for balance among them. But what does it mean to balance so many priorities? For instance, we may strive for balance between work and social activities. But there will be times when our goal of deep gratification in work requires us to disengage from social activities. We'll never strike that deal or get that dream job if we don't allow for some purposeful imbalance. On the other hand, there will be times when family or friends must take full priority over work. I just read an article about George Lucas, the *Star Wars* mogul, who took a decade off from filmmaking to raise his three kids. Such enforced, temporary imbalances can ultimately lead to greater balance—when we pull back and consider the big picture.

The fully lived life is usually characterized by both richness and lopsidedness. As leading mind-body expert Joan Borysenko recently said, "The only time we achieve a perfect state of balance is when we're dead."

That is why our approach to self-nurture must not be based on external rules or idyllic fantasies. I tell my patients to proceed with certain qualities of mind and heart: awareness rather than impulsiveness; gentleness rather than militance; flexibility rather than rigidity; desire rather than obligation.

This book focuses on key areas of women's lives that can cause dissatisfaction, stress, and pain. My goal—and I have not seen this set forth elsewhere—is to help women identify the areas that cause them the most distress, and to provide practical ways they can better care for themselves in each one. The sum of these realms is the sum of any woman's complex makeup. Women who learn self-nurture in each of these realms are saluting their own uniqueness.

The exercises in this book are offered in the spirit of self-exploration, to help you recognize and build your discoverable strengths. My wish is that you will find the inner resources, skills, desires, vulnerabilities, and resilience you never knew you had. As the Portuguese poet Fernando Pessoa once wrote, "In every corner of my soul there is an altar to a different God."

SELF-NURTURE: REDISCOVER YOUR APPETITE FOR LIFE

Self-Nurture is a yearlong stress manager for women. It offers specific guidance for handling the stresses that plague you, but the goal of every exercise and method is self-nurturance. It is a practical book, mapping greater awareness and self-care from one season to the next.

I offer this book as a balm for today's overextended, underappreciated, self-esteem-challenged women. While so many of us present smart, tough fronts to the world, we still suffer from grave insecurities and unfulfilled dreams. Psychiatrist Alexander Lowen once commented that we can only rise up if we allow ourselves to let down, and women who self-nurture will rise up with renewed strength and confidence. In a fascinating study, George Solomon found that patients with full-blown AIDS who "withdrew to nurture the self" remained miraculously healthy for extended periods of time. The same applies to those of us seeking mind-body health. Taking time for creative play and spiritual sustenance is medicine for body and soul. It restores meaning to days otherwise filled with hard work and daunting responsibilities.

Self-Nurture will be your exploratory map for living life to the fullest. In a recent interview, Diane Keaton was asked, "Given what you know from your own particular life, what would you pass on to your young daughter at this moment?" Her answer was passionate. "It would be great if she had a huge huge huge appetite for life. I really wish that for her. I hope that she embraces it enormously—every aspect of it. Headstrong. I hope that she is brave and curious and excited and interested, because that will pull her through."

Keaton's remark touches on the essence of my goal as a teacher of self-nurturance. As you take this book's journey, my fervent hope is that you can recapture your bravery, curiosity, and excitement—your huge appetite for life.

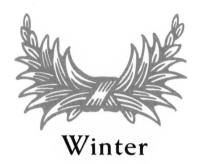

Winter

Primal Self-Care

2

MIND-BODY NURTURE:

THE BASICS

RECENTLY, A GOOD FRIEND, a bright, resourceful woman, told me why she was at the end of her tether. She was having a rough pregnancy; her mother was repeatedly returning to the hospital for treatment of a mysterious infection associated with her sudden recurrence of cancer; she was afflicted with writer's block trying to complete her master's thesis; she and her husband were about to relocate from New York to Los Angeles so he could get work as an actor; they had two hundred dollars left in their bank account; and their tiny sports car, used mainly to shuttle her mother to and from the hospital, was impounded due to late payments. The only solace they could find—no small comfort in the midst of this madness—was that neither she nor her husband had a terminal disease. As she ran down the list of troubles, oddly enough we found ourselves doubled over. When so many stressful events converge so preposterously, laughter is often the only means of maintaining your sanity.

While laughing with a friend over major stressors is real medicine, we need more than laughter when the real world keeps intruding with the message that we must somehow cope. We need specific skills for relaxation, coping, and spiritual sustenance.

Why does stress get the better of us? Why do we seem to lack creativity and vitality? In my decade of experience working with women—whether they have suffered from burnout, low self-esteem, marital conflict, loneliness, financial pressure, or chronic medical problems—the fundamental problem is not that we lack coping skills or relaxation techniques. Most of us do lack knowledge of these methods, but, more fundamentally, we're missing a commitment to ourselves that is rooted in compassion.

We lack the energy and initiative to solve problems *when we're so busy working and taking care of others that we neglect ourselves.* We lose commitment to a relaxation practice when *we don't feel entitled even to twenty minutes each day for our own well-being.* We set aside creative pursuits *because we internalize negative messages about our talents, or view artistic endeavors as one more drain on our crowded schedules.* And we lose heart *when our spiritual growth takes a backseat to duty and obligation.* In other words, our inability to self-nurture becomes a roadblock to all our efforts to manage stress, enhance health and energy, develop creativity, and cultivate soul.

Each upcoming chapter offers methods for self-nurture organized by different themes, and each thematic focus is broken down into four steps, one each for nurturing, the body, mind, emotions, and self/spirit. Here's what you will find in the four steps within each chapter:

- **Step 1: Nurture the Body.** Includes relaxation approaches, such as meditations and guided imagery. For instance, women with tumultuous relationships with husbands or partners may benefit from quiet meditation with a prayerful focus word; this practice fosters a sense of stillness. Women with severe anxiety about their body image can practice "progressive muscle relaxation" to reacquaint themselves with their bodies and loosen chronic muscular tensions.
- **Step 2: Nurture the Mind.** Centers on the use of "cognitive restructuring," a technique to help challenge negative thought patterns— the inner voices that help fuel anxiety, despair, and self-loathing. Replacing these thoughts with kinder and more realistic assessments is a form of mind-nurture. Negative thoughts, such as "I'm fat and I'll never feel good about my body," "I'll never amount to anything," "My husband is no longer attracted to me," and "I'm a horrible mother," can hound us into full-blown depression. We can restructure these thoughts based on a relentless truth-seeking analysis. After using the stepwise process I teach, one woman turned the negative thought "I'm a horrible mother" into the more affirmative "I'm actually a very good mother who has tried to attain perfection and fallen short in my all-too-critical eyes."
- **Step 3: Nurture the Emotions.** Includes practices of emotional awareness, expression, and communication. I use a specific ap-

proach to journal writing—exploring the depths of an issue or life event, past or present—as one way to practice awareness and expression. Communicating emotions also requires practice, and in many chapters I include methods for taking care of your emotional self in the context of your relationships, work, and creative activities.

- **Step 4: Nurture the Self/Spirit.** Involves making commitments to various parts of yourself (i.e., "I will take my creative self to a movie or museum every week," "I will honor my sexual self by letting my needs be known") or other ways to realize and enact kindnesses toward the self. You will also find imagery exercises and affirmations—positive statements or self-styled prayers said inwardly—that cultivate control, self-confidence, and inner peace.

Within each of the four steps, I offer a range of customized mind-body practices. To ground you in these techniques, and so I don't repeat basic instructions in each chapter, I will orient you to the basic mind-body practices here in this chapter. This will enable you to move easily through each chapter, to make these practices your own, to tailor them to each theme and to your individual needs.

Pathways to Relaxation

If self-nurturance is the soul of mind-body practice, relaxation is the heart. Relaxation techniques, ranging from meditation to progressive muscle relaxation to yoga, are all designed to elicit our inborn "relaxation response." While studying transcendental meditation (TM) in the 1970s, my colleague and mentor, Herbert Benson, M.D., discovered the physiologic changes associated with deep meditation: reduced heart rate, blood pressure, and oxygen consumption; slackened muscular tensions; raised skin temperature; and altered brain-wave patterns. He observed this set of changes not only when people practiced TM, but when they practiced virtually any established method of relaxation. Dr. Benson recognized that we all have the capacity to elicit these physiologic shifts, which occur in tandem with a calm mental state.

Benson named this becalmed mind-body state the "relaxation response." He viewed it as biology's answer to the fight-or-flight response—the set of changes that occur when we experience threat, danger, or acute stress. We've all experienced "fight or flight"—that adrenaline-driven state of anxiety or aggression characterized by a pounding heart, sweaty hands and brow, and the muscular readiness either to do battle or flee the scene. Indeed, fight or flight is part of our historical and genetic endowment, preserved through evolution as our psychobiological response to any threat to life and limb. Our prehistoric ancestors, the hunter-gatherers, were threatened by saber-toothed tigers, and through the course of history the threats have changed from wildlife to warrior nations to workaday pressures.

In today's world we respond to a mammogram or a boss's tirade much the way our predecessors reacted to tigers. Then and now, we "come down" from an acute state of high anxiety or aggression through a set of mind-body shifts. During fight or flight, our sympathetic nervous systems pump out stress hormones and our bodies are readied for action. Once the threat is gone, our sympathetic nervous systems decelerate: anxiety and aggression are eased, heart rate slows, blood pressure drops, and the brain waves move into a "calm" frequency range—the relaxation response.

In the modern world, the problem for most of us—men and women—is chronic stress, in which accumulating pressures, role demands, strained relationships, and financial difficulties leave us in a perpetual state of fight or flight. It's as if we were constantly being pursued by dangerous animals. Chronic stress can trigger continually high levels of stress hormones (for example, adrenaline and cortisol) that produce elevated blood pressure or heart rate, increased oxygen consumption, weakened immune systems, and other physiologic imbalances that eventually lead to symptoms or even full-blown diseases.

Most of us have had one or another stress-related disorder—the migraines, tension headaches, low back pain, hypertension, or auto-immune conditions we can directly link to traumas or periods of overwhelming stress. Dr. Benson has shown that by deliberately and regularly eliciting the relaxation response, we can use this natural mechanism to counter the effects of chronic stress on mind and body.

In the short term, eliciting the relaxation response produces nearly instant results—plummeting anxiety levels and the relief of physical tensions accompanied by a calmer physiology. When women practice relaxation on a daily basis, the long-term benefits are even more pronounced. They remain on an even keel for extended periods of time and are better able to cope with stress and fear, whether at work, behind the wheel of a car, or in a doctor's waiting room. In a matter of weeks, they also notice the alleviation of physical symptoms such as chronic headaches, back pain, and fatigue commonly caused by stress. In our research, we have demonstrated that regular relaxation results in a 57 percent reduction in the severe symptoms of PMS. We've also shown that menopausal women experience a significant decrease in depression and anxiety, not to mention a 28 percent reduction in the intensity of hot flashes.

There are numerous ways to elicit the relaxation response. The following section offers a short course on eight methods of relaxation. You will find these methods variously mentioned throughout the book, in some cases tailored for a particular need or issue regarding self-nurture. Refer back to this section whenever you need to remind yourself of these relaxation techniques; eventually, you won't need to.

First, a few simple guidelines when you practice any method for eliciting the relaxation response:

- Find a quiet place. Sitting in a comfortable chair is preferable, since you are less likely to fall asleep than when lying down. (If sitting is uncomfortable, lying down is fine; just monitor your tendency to drift into slumber.)
- Choose a regular time of day. For many women, the early morning is best, but there are no rules in this regard. It is best, however, to stick with one time; a sense of ritual keeps your commitment strong. Protect your relaxation time—let family or others know that you don't want to be interrupted for any nonemergency circumstances.
- There is no set time for relaxation, but most people take between 15 and 25 minutes; some sit for as long as 45 minutes to an hour. The average time, 20 to 25 minutes, is a good goal; it may also depend on the audiotape you may use as a guide. (See the appendix for a list of audiotapes.) Once-a-day practice is usually sufficient, though women who are particularly stressed surely may benefit from doing it twice a day.

I suggest that you sample all, or at least many, of the relaxation techniques that follow. Breath focus, the first method discussed, is a good place to start, and it is commonly used as an induction to other approaches. As you try out the different methods, you'll soon come to decide how you wish to spend the 15 to 25 minutes you set aside for relaxation. You may find you want to start with the breath focus for 5 minutes, then expend the rest of your time on, for example, the body scan or progressive muscle relaxation. Settle on a method that works best for you, but be flexible enough to mix, match, and change approaches when a particular technique no longer meets your needs.

Breath Focus

The goal of breath-focus relaxation is to shift from tense, shallow chest breathing to deep, relaxed abdominal breathing. During times of high stress or anxiety, our natural tendency is to hold our breaths. When the tension is chronic, we become shallow breathers, barely filling our lungs. As women, many of us were taught from an early age to hold in our stomachs, since our culture's concept of beauty revolves around the proverbial flat tummy. If we continuously tighten our stomach muscles, we lose the capacity to let the diaphragm move downward when we breathe. It's the descending diaphragm, that sheath of muscle separating the chest cavity from the abdominal cavity, that makes ample room for our lungs to fill during inhalation. But we must let our abdomens expand so the diaphragm can drop down, allowing oxygen to fill the bottom of our lungs. Otherwise, our bodies remain in a state of alarm, robbed of optimal oxygen. In turn, our anxiety levels surge, our breathing becomes even more shallow, and we get trapped in a vicious cycle of mental and physiologic tension.

Breath focus breaks the vicious cycle. The practice is simple:

- Take a normal breath. Don't change any aspect of how you breathe; simply take note of your breathing.
- Now take a deep, slow breath. Let the air come through your nose and move deeply into your lower belly. Take note of how your belly expands when you take such a deep breath; make no effort to limit this expansion. Then breathe out through your mouth.
- Take one normal breath, then one slow, deep abdominal breath. Alternate normal and deep breaths several times. As you do so, let

yourself become aware of how you feel on each inhalation and each exhalation. Compare and contrast the sensations associated with your normal breathing and your conscious deep breathing. Do you notice that your normal breathing is constricted? Does the deep breathing help you to relax?

- Now take time to practice deep breathing. Let the inhalations expand your belly. Now, on long, slow exhalations, allow yourself to sigh. Repeat this process for several minutes.

- For another 10 minutes or so, add another element to your practice. When you inhale, imagine that the air traveling in through your nose or mouth carries with it a sense of peace and calm. On the exhalation, imagine that the air traveling out of your nose or mouth carries out tension and anxiety. You may even wish to say these words silently to yourself on the inhalation: "Breathing in peace and calm." And, on the exhalation: "Breathing out tension and anxiety."

- Continue to focus on your deep breathing, letting in peace and calm, letting go of tension and anxiety. You may complete this entire process in about 20 minutes.

Body Scan

We all carry tension in different parts of our bodies, though often we are hardly aware of the muscle spasms present in the scalp, jaw, throat, chest, stomach, or pelvis. We hold stress, anxiety, or anger in varying muscular patterns, but the body scan relaxation practice can help anyone, regardless of where you carry tension or emotional distress. During the body scan, we close our eyes and "scan" our bodies with the mind's eye, becoming aware of muscular tensions. We then use breath awareness to focus on these tensions and to gradually let them go.

The body scan provides an opportunity to explore sensations in parts of your body you don't normally pay much attention to. You'll discover tensions and feelings you didn't know existed, and with practice you'll find yourself able to release the strain and pressure on different muscle groups with a simple awareness of your breath moving into and out of these areas.

The body scan practice involves several simple steps:

- Pay attention to your breathing. Allow your stomach to rise as you inhale, and to slowly fall back down as you exhale. Take some time to breath deeply before you begin the body scan.
- First concentrate on your forehead. As you breathe in, notice the muscles of your forehead. Become aware of any muscle tension in your forehead. As you breathe out, let go of any muscle tension you find there. Continue this practice—awareness of forehead tension on the in-breath, letting go of forehead tension on the out-breath—for several slow, deep breaths.
- For the remainder of the body scan exercise, repeat this process: Concentrate on any muscle tension in a particular body area as you inhale. Now, as you exhale, use your consciousness to loosen and release that tension. (Some people find it useful to imagine the breath traveling into the particular body part, then traveling out as they exhale. As the breath leaves the area, they visualize the muscles slackening, as if the departing breath carries the tension away with it.) Make certain to take slow, deep breaths, perhaps noticing how your stomach rises as you inhale and falls as you exhale. Now move down gradually and repeat the process in these bodily areas:
- Scan your eyes and the muscles around them.
- Scan your mouth and jaw. You may notice that your jaw drops a bit as you exhale, letting go of tension in that area.
- Scan your throat and neck.
- Scan your back, all the way from the top of your spine down to your tailbone.
- Scan your shoulders.
- Scan your upper arms, from where they meet your shoulders down to the elbows.
- Scan your lower arms, from the elbows down and including your hands and fingers.
- Scan your chest.
- Scan your stomach.
- Scan your pelvis and buttocks.
- Scan your upper legs.
- Scan your lower legs, ankles, and feet.
- As your body scan relaxation comes to a close, do a mental check on your entire body, from your head down to your toes. If you no- tice remaining areas of muscular tension, let yourself become

aware of them as you breathe in. Let go of these muscle tensions as you breathe out.

Some people have difficulty with body scanning, finding it too abstract to try and "feel" body parts they are unaccustomed to feeling (eyes, for example). If this applies to you, progressive muscle relaxation may be more effective.

Progressive Muscle Relaxation

Progressive muscle relaxation (PMR) adds an important new element to the body scan practice. Instead of simply using mental focus and breathing to relax tense muscle groups, we consciously increase these tensions before letting go. This practice concretizes the effort to relax muscles, intensifying the sensations of both tension and release. For some people, this enhances the sense that they're able to slacken tight muscles and brings a refreshing feeling of relaxation to the entire body. Women with chronic pain might find that PMR increases discomfort by calling so much attention to the part of the body that causes suffering. But people who have trouble sensing or relaxing tense areas may find this highly active, concrete exercise to be most effective. (Some people prefer to practice PMR lying down.) The steps involved in PMR are similar to those of the body scan, with the key variation of actual tightening of muscles:

- Pay attention to your breathing. Allow your stomach to rise as you inhale and to come back down as you exhale. Take several deep breaths before you begin.
- Now concentrate on your forehead. Consciously tighten the muscles of your forehead while counting slowly from 1 to 5. Hold your forehead muscles as tight as you can for the duration of this count. Then let go of your tense forehead muscles while taking a slow, deep breath. Notice your stomach rise as you inhale, then come back down as you exhale. Now do this again: Tighten your forehead muscles for a count of 5; release those muscles as you take a slow, deep breath.
- For the remainder of the PMR exercise, repeat this process: Move down the body, and tighten the muscles in a particular body area for a count of 1 to 5; then *release that tension as you take a slow,*

deep breath. Repeat this process—tightening and releasing as you breathe—twice for each bodily area. Now move gradually down the body and practice PMR in these bodily areas:

- Tighten and release the muscles around your eyes by squeezing your eyes tightly shut, then gently opening them.
- Tighten and release your jaw.
- Tighten and release your neck muscles by lowering your chin to your chest, then gently bringing it back up.
- Tighten your right shoulder, raising it as high as you can. Let go of the tension.
- Tighten your right upper arm, from the shoulder to the elbow, by flexing your arm as tightly as you can. Let go of the tension.
- Tighten and release your right forearm.
- Tighten your right hand into a fist; release.
- Take a moment now to notice if your right arm feels different from your left arm. Is your right arm more relaxed?
- Repeat this process on your left side: tightening and releasing your left shoulder, upper arm, forearm, and hand in the same manner you did on your right side.
- Tighten and release your back, all the way from the top of your spine down to your tailbone, by trying to get your shoulderblades to meet in back.
- Tighten and release your chest.
- Tighten and release your abdomen.
- Tighten and release your pelvis and buttocks.
- Tighten and release your right upper leg.
- Tighten and release your right lower leg.
- Tighten your right foot by flexing it; let go of the tension.
- Take a moment now to notice if your right leg and foot feels different from your left leg and foot. Is your right leg and foot more relaxed?
- Tighten and release your left upper leg.
- Tighten and release your left lower leg.
- Tighten your left foot by flexing it; let go of the tension.
- Once you finish tightening and releasing all the muscle groups, do a mental check on your entire body, from your head down to your toes. If you notice remaining areas of tension, tense those muscles

for a count of 1 to 5; then let go of these muscles as you take slow, deep breaths.

Meditation

The practice of meditation, at least twenty-five hundred years old, comes to us from both Eastern and Western spiritual traditions, from Hinduism to Buddhism to Judaism. Each tradition has its own singular philosophy and technique, though certain threads are common in virtually all meditative practices. Typically, meditation involves a turning inward of our attention, a repetitive focus on breathing and a simple word, phrase, or prayer. Many spiritual traditions also encourage the meditator to take a nonjudgmental attitude toward any thoughts or feelings that arise during practice.

It is not necessary to adopt a spiritual attitude or religious philosophy in order to practice meditation in a meaningful way. Of course, many meditators bring their beliefs into practice, and others who have no religious or spiritual affiliation still enjoy using a focus word or phrase that has special meaning or resonance. Indeed, you may choose a word or phrase to use in meditation that is secular (e.g., "Let it Be" or "Peace") or religious (i.e., "Hail Mary" for Christians, "Shalom," for Jews.) For the following simple instruction, I offer the old Sanskrit mantra, *Ham Sah*. (*Ham* means "I am"; *Sah* means "That.") Many patients use it because the sounds comfortably reflect the sensations of breathing and letting go. Feel free to substitute other words or phrases.

Take note: Many of us have racing or wandering minds. The purpose of meditation is not to control this tendency rigidly. Rather, meditation gives us a gentle way to shift from intrusive thoughts and feelings to a focus on our breath and the repetition of a simple phrase. When anxious fantasies, memories, or worries abound, we can accept their inevitability and recognize them for what they are—just the nagging mind. Then, we can return to our focus on breath and phrase, and return again and again when such thoughts arise. Remember, meditation is a process without a fixed goal, and it should not be your intention to do it perfectly—just to do it. Begin by setting aside ten minutes for each session, then gradually work yourself up to twenty minutes or more.

Meditation practice is not complicated:

- Find a comfortable place to sit and close your eyes. Starting with the number 10, silently count down to zero, breathing in and out on each count. Notice that your breathing may slow as you count down.
- Now as you breath in, say the word *Ham* (pronounced *Haam*) silently to yourself. Imagine the sound reverberating in your mind, like the *hmmm* feeling you get when you sink into a hot bath. As you exhale, concentrate on the word *Sah* (pronounced *Saah*) in your mind, like a sigh. Do this for several moments. If your attention wanders, gently bring it back to *Ham* as you inhale, and *Sah* as you exhale.
- Continue to note your breathing. As you inhale, pause for a few seconds. As you exhale, pause for a few seconds. Let your breathing slow as you think *Ham* on the inhale, *Sah* on the exhale.
- If your mind starts to wander, return to *Ham Sah*. Stay as focused as you can on your breathing and these words. And don't judge yourself as you meditate. If thoughts or feelings intrude, neither encourage them nor push them away. Just quietly resume your breathing and repeating *Ham Sah*.
- As time for meditation comes to a close, continue to be aware of your breathing, but start to be aware of where you are, the sounds around you, where you are sitting. When ready, slowly open your eyes, look down for a few moments, and get up gradually.

Mindfulness

Mindfulness is both a meditation and a philosophy, rooted in ancient principles of Tibetan Buddhism. Mindfulness as a daily practice grounds us in the present, and its philosophy teaches that the present is the only realm in which we are capable of joy and fulfillment. Jon Kabat-Zinn, founder and director of the Stress Reduction Clinic of the University of Massachusetts, arguably America's leading teacher of mindfulness, reminds us that much of our suffering can be traced to our "stuckness" in either the past or the future. We may be haunted by regrets, painful memories, or unresolved relationships. Or we may be trapped by our own fearful anticipation of disasters awaiting us tomorrow, next month, or next year. Living in memories or thoughts of the future, we become unaware and unappreciative of what is happening in the here and now. In other words, we become mindless.

The antidote to mind*less*ness is mind*ful*ness. Mindfulness as a way of life means nourishing our capacity to be in the present, which engenders gratitude for the wonders we experience through our senses, emotions, and intellects. Mindfulness meditation is a specific practice that enables us to become mindful in daily life—not just during the meditation itself. The simple prescriptions of mindfulness meditation can literally be transferred to our daily activities, enabling us to bring here-and-now awareness to all our activities—creative work, cooking a meal, making love, cleaning house, eating, playing with children, taking a walk in the park. In my own life and the lives of many patients, one consistently useful practice is the "mindful walk," in which we stroll along quietly, with total moment-to-moment sensory awareness of our environment—be it the sounds and sights of a city street or the smells and views of a country road. The combination of mindfulness and exercise can both ground and energize us in the midst of stressful times.

Use the mindfulness meditation to build awareness, peacefulness, the capacity for pleasure, and gratitude into your daily existence. I will first present guidelines for the basic mindfulness meditation, which is similar to the basic meditation but with a particular emphasis on grounding in the moment. Then, I will illustrate how you can transfer this ability to daily life in the form of a mindful activity—eating an orange. (Of course, being a dedicated chocoholic, I actually teach this to my patients by having them eat a Hershey's Kiss mindfully.)

Mindfulness meditation

- Begin the same way you would with basic meditation, becoming aware of and focusing on your breathing. You may wish to use a focus word or phrase, but for mindfulness meditation this is not necessary. Use one if it feels comfortable to do so. Without a focus word or phrase, simply concentrate on the sensations of your breathing—your belly as it rises and falls, the air as it enters your nostrils and leaves your mouth.
- You may notice thoughts continuously arising, perhaps in the form of worries, anxieties, fears, hopes, or fantasies. This is a natural process of the mind. So as you sit in stillness, your body in a

state of quiet and relaxation, watch each thought as it comes and goes. Be exquisitely conscious—mindful—of the process of thinking. Witness how your thoughts are continually shifting—subtly changing, moving, dissolving.

- When you notice that you've been carried away in a stream of associations, or in a stream of thoughts, just observe that this has happened. Without judgment, without being hard on yourself, gently return to awareness of your breath, being aware of the breath in the foreground, while the thoughts may continue in the background. The breath is the most natural way to center yourself and be anchored in the present moment.
- For the remaining time, keep your breathing in the foreground of your awareness. As if you were a silent witness, observe any sensations in the body, thoughts in the mind, or sounds in the environment. Be aware of these sensations, thoughts, or sounds without fighting them or clinging to them. Keep returning to the breath as the anchor of your awareness. As you complete this mindfulness meditation, know that the benefits can expand, enabling you to bring full attention to whatever you do during the rest of the day. Now, at your own pace, bring your awareness back to your surroundings.

Mindful activity

- Get yourself a nice plump orange. Eat it with full awareness of every movement, bite, and sensation. First, peel the orange. Be aware of the smell of the orange and what it looks like as you peel off the rind. Notice how your fingers feel as they dig into the rind, and recognize your anticipation as you tear and twirl it away from the surface of the orange itself. Slowly separate the sections, observing their shape, recognizing the sounds and feel of the entire process. As you take your first bite of an orange section, attend to every sensation on your lips, tongue, the roof of your mouth. Notice how tart the flavor is at first, then, gradually, how sweet. Feel the squirting juice on the inside of your mouth. Eat slowly, savoring each bite and fully receiving every taste sensation. (If you're feeling a bit decadent, try this with a Hershey's Kiss.)
- Take as much time as you need to complete this exercise. It must be done very slowly.

Guided Imagery

Mind pictures, dreams, visions—they have long been the basis for healing rituals in cultures worldwide. But science has recently begun to
prove that visual imagery is not just a phenomenon of mind, it is also a
phenomenon of body. All you have to do is visualize yourself licking a
slice of lemon, and the tiny jets of saliva released in the back of your
mouth tell you that imagery has physiologic consequences.

Guided imagery was first popularized in the 1970s as a potential
treatment for cancer patients, who were encouraged to imagine their
cancer cells being eaten up by vigorous immune cells or vengeful chemotherapy drugs. While there has been no definitive evidence that these
approaches led to regression of cancers, there *has* been evidence that
guided imagery, or visualization, as it is also known, can enhance immune function, reduce the side effects of chemotherapy, and alleviate
pain.

Most important, certain types of imagery can elicit the relaxation response. I use several imagery exercises that my patients find helpful. In
one, you see yourself taking a walk on a deserted beach; another has you
strolling a path toward a mountain stream; yet another has you slowly
descending into a luxurious hot bath. In the chapters ahead, I recommend these and other imagery exercises. I will provide scripts you may
use as guides, or you may order the imagery tapes read by myself or my
colleagues (see the appendix). I also tailor guided imagery exercises for
specific areas of your life where you need more self-nurture. When you
project relaxing, uplifting, emotional, or spiritually laden images on the
screen of your own mind, you engage in a powerful exercise in self-
awareness and self-nurture.

The following is a basic template for the practice of guided imagery,
a method you can use for any type of visualization:

- Find a quiet place where you can sit in a comfortable position.
  Close your eyes and take several slow, deep, cleansing breaths.
- Now go in your mind to a special place that you love, a place where
  you have felt relaxed or know you would feel relaxed. It can be a favorite vacation spot; your parents' or grandparents' backyard; a
  place you have seen in the movies. It does not matter what environment you choose, as long as it makes you feel at peace.

- Now spend time in this peaceful place, seeing yourself sitting or standing in one spot, or moving along. Take in the sounds, smells, and views all around you.
- Focus on colors and shapes. If you are outdoors, note the color of the sky, the shape of the clouds. See the whole expanse of sky or sand or grass or forest or stream. If you're in your grandmother's backyard, see the scene in its entirety. What does the lawn or terrace look like? Visualize the trees, shrubbery, fences, or outdoor chairs that were part of the environment you remember.
- Focus on smells. If you're on a beach, smell the ocean or the suntan lotion. If you're in your best friend's house, conjure up the aromas that were present in the living room, the cooking odors from the kitchen, the fragrance of grass and trees in the yard. Savor the fresh air smells deep in the forest, by your favorite babbling brook.
- Focus on sounds. Listen to the ocean waves breaking; the sound of your grandmother's voice; the gurgling of water across rocks in the brook.
- Focus on movement. The movement of clouds or water or seagulls or cars. If you wish, see yourself moving—walking on the sand inspecting seashells; traipsing through high grass in the backyard; bouncing from rock to rock in the babbling brook.
- Focus on sensations. The feeling of salty ocean air on your skin; the grass tickling your naked feet; the slippery surfaces of the rocks as you step along in that brook.
- Allow yourself to become totally absorbed in the sensual aspects of these images, all in a place where you feel comfortable, at home, at peace. If your sense of peace is interrupted by anxious or disturbing thoughts or images, observe them. Then gently return to the specific sights, smells, and sensations that surround you.

Autogenic Training

Autogenic training uses verbal suggestions in what amounts to a form of progressive relaxation for the body. Developed in the 1930s by the German physician Johannes Schultz, the method relies upon verbal suggestions, called "orientations," as a subtle form of self-hypnosis. During autogenic training, you bypass your conscious mind in order to instruct your body to relax. The secret behind autogenic training may lie in the fact that our minds so often obstruct our bodies' efforts to calm down; by sidestepping the mind, we set up more direct communication with the body. The training is therefore a great choice for women who have trouble with meditation, mindfulness, or breath focus—in other words, women with wildly racing minds.

• Find a comfortable place to sit, and take a few slow, deep, cleansing breaths.

   Focus on the sensations of your breath; imagine it rolling in and out like ocean waves. As you imagine waves of relaxation flowing through your body—your chest and shoulders, your arms and back, your hips and legs—silently repeat this phrase: "My breath is calm and effortless . . . calm and effortless. . . ." Do this for several minutes.

   Focus on your arms and hands. As you breathe deeply, repeat in your mind slowly and clearly, "My arms are heavy and warm. Warmth is flowing through my arms into my wrists, hands, and fingers." Focus for a few minutes on these thoughts and on the feelings in your arms and hands.

   Next, bring your focus to your legs. Imagine warmth and heaviness flowing from your arms down into your legs. Think to yourself, "My legs are becoming heavy and warm. Warmth is flowing down through my feet into my toes. My legs and feet are heavy and warm."

   Scan your body for points of tension, then let those places go limp, your muscles relaxed. Notice how heavy, warm, and limp your body has become. Think, "All my muscles are letting go. I'm getting more and more relaxed."

   Finally, take a deep breath, feeling the air fill your lungs and move down into your abdomen. As you breathe out, think, "I am calm . . . I am calm. . . ." Continue doing this for several minutes, as you become aware of the peacefulness throughout your body.

   End the session by counting to 3, then take a deep breath and exhale with each number. Open your eyes and give yourself a few moments to return to awareness of your surroundings. Stand up slowly and stretch before you resume your regular activities.

- Allow yourself to get lost in the sound of your own voice as you repeat each statement clearly and slowly in your mind. Listen to the words and follow their lead as you breathe deeply.

Yoga

Another powerful approach is yoga, the three-thousand-year-old practice based on Indian spiritual teachings, a blend of physical postures, meditation, and deep breathing. The extensive variety of yogic systems, practices, and postures all involve *pranayamas,* or breathing purifications; asanas, or stretching postures, as well as meditations that foster inner tranquility. Yogic exercises are gentle ways of moving, stretching, and breathing for relaxation and reinvigoration of mind and body. As a form of meditation in motion, yoga carries unique benefits that more "passive" methods may not yield—mainly, the vitalizing movement of energy through the body.

Because everyone's body is so distinct, yoga should be individualized. Most experts in yoga believe, rightly, I think, that the discipline is best learned with a yoga teacher who can guide the student to poses and practices that suit his unique physical "personality." Also, given the variety of yogic systems, it makes sense for you to sample different approaches and teachers before settling on one. I have found a few books that are useful, offering easy-to-follow poses, but they are best used in tandem with a class. Among them are *Yoga for Wellness* by Gary Kraftsow; *Yoga for Women* by Paddy O'Brien; *Complete Stretching* by Maxine Tobias; and a chapter on yoga by my former colleague Margaret Ennis in *The Wellness Book* by Herbert Benson, M.D., and Eileen Stuart, R.N.

Mini-Relaxations

I refer to mini-relaxations as "the perfect portable stress managers," because they are the only relaxation exercise you can safely and secretly practice in public. You can do a mini-relaxation in your car, in the middle of a meeting, in the thick of a difficult interaction with a colleague or loved one. My patients swear by "minis," as I call them, because they can help them out of any jam, anytime. Whether you're a mother having a hard day with your toddler, an executive in the eye of an organizational storm, or a wife in the midst of marital trouble, you can rely on minis to calm down and reclaim your center.

Mini-relaxations are short-form versions of the breath-focus meditation. They allow you rapidly to shift from shallow chest breathing to deep abdominal (diaphragmatic) breathing in the batting of an eyelash. I teach four different methods of mini-relaxation, which, in my experience, are the easiest and most reliable ones. The first version enables you to make the breathing shift, and it is useful initially to practice it lying down, since the prone position makes you more aware of your breathing patterns. Otherwise, you can practice minis whenever and wherever you wish—standing, lying, sitting, running, or, for that matter, rollerskating. Here are the four versions:

Mini-Relaxation—Version 1

Sit or, preferably, lie down in a comfortable position. Take a deep, slow breath. Place a hand on your abdomen, just on top of your belly button. Allow your abdomen to rise about an inch as you inhale. As you exhale, notice that your abdomen falls about an inch. Also notice that your chest rises slightly as your abdomen rises.

Become aware of your diaphragm moving down as you inhale, back up as you exhale. Remember that it's impossible to breath abdominally if your diaphragm does not move down. And your diaphragm won't move down if you keep your stomach tight. So soften your stomach muscles.

If you find this difficult, try breathing through your nose and out your mouth. Attend to the sensations of abdominal breathing for several breaths, or as long as you desire.

Mini-Relaxation—Version 2

Make the shift from chest breathing to deep abdominal breathing. Count down from 10 to zero, taking one complete breath—one inhalation, one exhalation—with each number. Thus, with your first abdominal breath, you say "ten" to yourself, with the next breath you say "nine," and so on. If you start to feel light-headed or dizzy, slow down your counting. When you get to zero, see how you are feeling. If you're feeling more relaxed, great. If not, try it again.

Mini-Relaxation—Version 3

Make the shift from chest breathing to deep abdominal breathing. As you inhale, count very slowly from 1 to 4. As you exhale, count slowly back down, from 4 to 1. Thus, as you inhale, you say silently to yourself, "One, two, three, four." As you exhale, you say silently to yourself, "Four, three, two, one." Do this for several breaths, or for as long as you wish.

Mini-Relaxation—Version 4

Make the shift from chest breathing to deep abdominal breathing. Use any of the other three methods as you breathe: simply breathe as you feel your stomach rise, and add a 10-to-0 count with each breath, or add a 1-to-4/4-to-1 count as you inhale and exhale. But this time, regardless of what method you use, pause for a few seconds after each in-breath. Pause again for a few seconds after each out-breath. Do this for several breaths, or for as long as you wish.

Mini-relaxations don't yield the same long-term benefits of the lengthier relaxation practices that require at least 15 minutes in solitude, but they can have pronounced short-term physiologic and psychologic effects. Physiologically, they improve oxygen exchange, lower heart rate and blood pressure. Psychologically, they enhance your perception of control, and they distract you from fear and pain, which makes them perfect stress managers when you are undergoing medical tests, procedures, or encounters with doctors. Some of my infertility patients have gotten through years of fertility treatments by constantly practicing minis.

I have patients with cancer, endometriosis, PMS, hot flashes, infertility, and other medical and psychological symptoms who use minis as frequently as a hundred times per day. We tend to hold our breath when we're stressed, which immediately sets the stage for that vicious cycle of anxiety, oxygen starvation, impoverished breathing, and ever-worsening levels of stress. Minis break the cycle quickly and efficiently, so use them liberally. The mini-relaxation is one stress manager for which you need little time, no money, no privacy, and only one portable asset—your lungs.

Among the other useful relaxation techniques that I recommend are hypnosis and biofeedback, although I do not teach them. Perhaps I haven't gravitated to hypnosis and biofeedback because they require another person, an expert, to "administer" the practice. While these methods are surely effective for many people, especially those with medical conditions, my focus has always been self-care—methods women can generally practice on their own, without anyone else's direction or control.

I suggest that you try the above methods as if you were at a Chinese buffet, sampling the fare and going back for second helpings of those you most enjoy. To the best of your ability, explore these approaches with imagination, a sense of freedom, and a lightness of being. Relaxation should not be a chore; it should, in fact, be the very essence of your commitment to self-nurture, a daily signifier of your care for yourself.

Relaxation means taking time to yourself, by yourself, and for yourself. You may not always want to stop what you are doing, shift gears, and move into another state of mind, so the initial push may feel like just another obligation in a busy day. But once you commit yourself to one method, or even to a lazy-Susan approach of varying methods, that sense of compulsion will fade.

Remember, you don't have to stick with one relaxation technique forever. A lot of women find that they practice different techniques to match their moods. You may even discover that depending on your physical state, one technique might work better than another. I don't normally do well with meditation; my mind can't seem to stay focused on a word or phrase. But a strange thing happened while I was pregnant with Sarah and went into labor at twenty-seven weeks. My doctor was able to stop the labor with medication and sent me home with strict instructions to stay in bed and relax. For all my mind-body training, this was no easy task. I tried several relaxation methods that had worked for me in the past, such as body scan and breath focus, but none of them made me feel less anxious about the risk of prematurely delivering Sarah. In desperation, I tried meditation. Since Sarah was due in late January, on the in-breath I recited, "We will make it," and on the out-breath, I said, "to January."

I repeated this meditation several times a day, and it truly helped calm me and made me feel more in control of the situation. Although some research has shown that relaxation techniques can stop premature labor, I can't say that this practice was responsible for delaying Sarah's delivery until January 9—and my doctor is convinced it was the drugs that made the difference. Ironically, after Sarah was born, I was once again unable to meditate!

If you find that a particular technique you'd previously found effective is suddenly not working, experiment with different techniques. Your preference may shift in response to the day of the week, your menstrual cycle, the lunar cycle . . . anything that can affect your mind, body, or soul.

Cognitive Restructuring: The Mind-Nurture Method

For just one day, try listening to the voices in your head. If you keep a rough record of the comments you make to yourself, you'll discover that the vast majority are negative in tone and content. In my experience with women who carefully monitor their thoughts, most find that 90 percent are negative. How many of us wake up in the morning, look in the mirror, and say, "How stunning!" "Great hair!" "Fabulous thighs!" "Smashing success in the world!"? Instead, we wake to withering self-criticisms, statements that we reiterate throughout the day. Perhaps the best analogy for our harsh, critical inner voice is that of the negative tape loop—a repetitive, nagging monologue of fearful or self-denigrating comments about ourselves, our bodies, our abilities, and our prospects for happiness.

We all have our own "greatest hits"—specific tracks of negative self-talk that we replay at the slightest provocation, or no provocation at all. And women in America have quite a number of collective greatest hits: "I'm fat," "I'll never amount to anything," "I'm a bad mother" are just a few.

These self-punishing thought patterns represent the foundation of our low self-esteem. They're like mental fuel for anxiety and depression: How could we not become anxious when we repeatedly tell ourselves what terrible things are about to happen? How could we not become depressed when we repeatedly tell ourselves that we're worthless and that our lot is hopeless?

Despite their horrific content and deleterious effects, such thoughts are hard to resist. Relentless, unfounded negative thoughts are like tobacco—they're addictive and they carry no health benefits. Indeed, they are so poisonous to our health and well-being that the cigarette analogy is not the least bit far-fetched: our nasty minds can make us sick. When faced with stress or challenge, the stream of negative self-talk only boosts the stress response, causing chronic states of fear or help-lessness that further disable our coping abilities. Over time, the psychological and physical effects may include cardiovascular disorders, immune dysfunction, and a worsening of stress-related symptoms, from headaches and back pain to asthma and autoimmune diseases like rheumatoid arthritis.

Cognitive restructuring, the central technique of cognitive therapy pioneered by psychologist Aaron Beck, is a form of mind-nurture that can free us from the punishing mind that holds us prisoner of our own echoing critical voices. The key to cognitive restructuring is not that we counter the nasty mind with the dreamy mind or the self-inflating mind. Rather, we defuse the punishing mind with a balanced, thoughtful, self-caring series of questions. These new questions can yield brand-new answers, from which we seek and often find a much deeper level of truth, one that guides us toward improvements in our relationships, work, and self-image. Cognitive restructuring bolsters self-esteem, not by having us attack others or fatten our own egos, but by building a realistic compassion for ourselves and others.

Cognitive therapy makes this process relatively simple and straight-forward. Four questions help us become aware of negative thought patterns, doggedly challenge their logic, and replace them with kinder and more realistic thoughts that enhance our well-being. Although cognitive restructuring is not complicated, it is not always easy, prompting us to explore more deeply our inner demons, childhood sources of negative thoughts, or current relationships that reinforce insecurity and self-doubt. The process helps us identify these sources and diffuse their power by labeling them for what they are: voices of the past or present that are usually groundless, exaggerated, or downright nonsensical.

- First, identify one common negative thought pattern, one tape loop that plays repeatedly in your head.
- Write down this negative tape loop as a sentence or two.
- Now, ask yourself these four questions about this negative thought:

  1. Does this thought contribute to my stress?
  2. Where did I learn this thought?
  3. Is this a logical thought?
  4. Is this thought true?

Before you can restructure an automatic negative thought, you must first honestly confront that thought, discover its origins and effects, and put it to the test of logic. That is the purpose of the four questions.

One of my patients, Lorraine, used the four questions to help her deal with constant negative thoughts regarding her relationship with her live-in mate, Mike. Whenever Lorraine became moody, and Mike did not immediately respond with loving support, Lorraine convinced herself that he was fed up and would soon leave her. It got to the point that whenever she would show or even experience unhappy emotion in Mike's presence, she immediately thought, "Mike's going to leave me because he can't take my mood swings."

Lorraine's answer to the first question, *Does this thought contribute to my stress?*, was clear: This thought was contributing to her stress on a daily basis. The second question was pivotal: *Where did this thought come from?* Lorraine's breakthrough came when she realized that her thoughts came from her relationship with her father. She had a troubled connection with him from early childhood; he became critical and distant whenever Lorraine was angry or blue. This created a powerful template in Lorraine's mind: Show a male figure you are unhappy and he will abandon you. Once she recognized the origins of her negative tape loop in her relationship with her father, Lorraine was able to start separating the shadows of the past from the reality of the present—her relationship with Mike. This was not a quick or an easy process, but her cognitive work was the positive turning point.

Question three deepened the process. *Was her thought logical?* No. Lorraine had no real evidence to support her belief that Mike would soon leave her. This helped defuse her fears, but it was not enough. Having debunked the logic behind her thought, Lorraine still needed to answer question four—was her thought ultimately true? It was true that Mike sometimes had difficulty when Lorraine became moody, and yes, he was perplexed by her fears of abandonment. But he loved her and was not considering leaving her due to these difficulties. This dynamic was indeed a problem in their relationship, but Lorraine's repetitive belief that she'd soon be abandoned had no basis in truth.

The final step in cognitive restructuring is to replace the negative thought with a kinder, more realistic assessment. Lorraine's restructuring was simple: "When I get moody, I fear abandonment due to my past with my father. Mike may get upset, but he reassures me that he is not leaving, and I believe him." From then on, whenever these fearful thoughts arose, Lorraine would take a deep breath, close her eyes, and say this to herself like a mantra.

Answering each of the four questions sets the stage for thought restructuring. To recap, first you need to recognize that your negative thought contributes to your stress. Second, determine the origins of your negative thought, which is so often the critical voice of someone from your past or present, or your own fear intruding. Third, use your rational mind to determine if your thought is even logical. And fourth, decide whether the thought contains any truth whatsoever, and characterize and assess its level of truth. (Question three on logic and question four on truth may overlap somewhat, but both are necessary. Sometimes a thought is illogical yet still has some truth, and sometimes it's logical but not absolutely true. For instance, it may not be logical to believe that your mother is harboring a grudge against you, but she may be anyway. Or it may be logical to think that your past difficulties taking scholastic tests means you're likely to fail your next exam, but that doesn't mean it's true.)

Once you have fully answered and explored the four questions, you can create your own restructured thought, which I recommend that you write down under the original negative thought. Refer to your restructured thought whenever the negative thought reemerges. You can even use it as a mantra in meditation, if you find it helpful.

It's easy to see how important cognitive work is to women's mental health and quality of life. If Lorraine had never restructured her thinking, had she continued for months or years to continuously fear abandonment, it's not hard to imagine that her feelings and behavior would eventually result in a serious breach in her relationship. Mike may eventually have gotten fed up listening to her baseless fears, since the underlying message would be that she couldn't trust him. Endlessly unchallenged negative thinking can sometimes lead to self-fulfilling prophecy.

When you practice the four questions and thought replacement, take time with your answers. Approach the process as you would a mindfulness meditation—with deep breaths and a keen awareness. You will discover surprising truths, strong emotions, and sharp insights into yourself and your loved ones. These realizations will help you to heal your relationships, rebuild your self-image, and markedly reduce your daily stress.

Emotional Expression: Keeping a Journal

Nurturing emotions should be an integral part of our broader efforts to self-nurture. Much of our stress originates from within, when anger or grief has us by the throat. Contrary to popular opinion, the answer is not to talk ourselves out of negative feelings, suppress them, or even to discharge them in explosive efforts to "ventilate." First, we need to accept the full range of emotions, our entire grand palette, and stop labeling them "negative." Grief, anger, and fear may be experienced as "negative," but they are also adaptive emotions that serve us well; they signal that something is wrong in our environment, or that a past trauma is still exerting its effects on our psyche. We need to listen to these feelings, accept their validity within ourselves (rather than wait for someone else to validate them), privately work through them, share them when appropriate, and resolve their effects on mind and body. When we don't nurture emotions in these ways, they accumulate in mind and body with potentially harmful effects on our psychological well-being. In some respects, depression is unexpressed sadness; anxiety is unexplored fear; and irritability is unresolved anger. Moreover, depression, anxiety, and irritability are commonly associated with the development of physical disorders ranging from immune dysfunctions to heart disease.

In my mind-body practice, one of the best ways to explore, express, and therefore nurture emotions is through journaling. Psychologist James W. Pennebaker of the University of Texas has conducted at least a dozen studies of people who write out their most painful thoughts and feelings for 20 minutes every day for four days. Unlike control subjects who write about trivial events, these people experience marked improvements in their psychological and physical well-being. They become less anxious and depressed, and they are physically healthier for as long as five months afterwards. Researchers at the University of North Dakota, using Pennebaker's writing technique, showed marked improvements in patients with asthma and arthritis, as compared to a control group. (The study was deemed significant enough to be published in 1999 in the *Journal of the American Medical Association*.) Dr. Pennebaker has also demonstrated that subjects who wrote about past traumas for four days had stronger T-lymphocytes—immune cells that extinguish disease agents—for a period of six weeks. Pennebaker has found that not only writing but also talking about past traumas or current stress can be healing.

I have followed Dr. Pennebaker's specific prescriptions for writing exercises that nurture emotions, freeing us from the strangling effect of unexplored feeling. They are as follows:

- Sit down with blank paper in front of you. (If you prefer using a computer, that's fine, too.) For 20 minutes, write nonstop about the most stressful event or ongoing problem you face in your daily life. If you believe your current problems are primarily the result of past events, write about the traumatic circumstances in your past. Don't worry about grammar or sentence structure. Write about what happened, and how you felt or feel about it. Don't stick exclusively to facts or to feelings—write about both. (Pure facts without feelings won't be liberating. Pure feeling with no facts won't help you to understand your experiences. This process involves both emotional catharsis and insight.)
- Repeat this 20-minute process for at least three or four days, and keep going for as long as a week if you find that the exercise continues to be fruitful. If you've covered one traumatic event or stressful circumstance, and there are other ones pressing, move on and explore them, as well.
- If you have a medical condition that causes emotional distress, write nonstop for 20 minutes about the most traumatic event or stressful aspect of this condition. Then follow the same guidelines above, and continue the exercise every day for at least three or four days.

This writing exercise is a fundamental approach I teach to help women nurture emotions in every area of their lives. As you move through the next seven chapters, you'll find that I apply this approach to varying issues and situations. You may write about painful emotions associated with relationships with family members or partners; strained friendships; a negative body image; sexual difficulties; money problems; health conditions; or spiritual distress. I will provide specific questions you can use as launchpads for nurturing emotions in each of these areas.

In my experience, such writing explorations can be remarkably helpful, and sometimes healing, as you acknowledge your wounds and free yourself from pent-up anger, fear, and sorrow. There's an uncanny alchemy about writing that is different from every other approach to catharsis and healing—including psychotherapy, talking to friends, and confessing to clergy.

A number of years ago, soon after I had heard about Pennebaker's work, a close friend of mine made an insulting remark about a deeply personal issue. I experienced his words as not only insensitive but downright cruel. Because I am usually loath to confront people, I never told my friend that he'd caused such anguish. As a result, I felt helplessly stuck with my rage and hurt. With no other option, I sat at my computer and ferociously wrote down my thoughts and feelings about my friend's comments—the circumstances in which he'd made them and the emotions they triggered. Then I considered why his statements had caused so much pain—exploring my own vulnerability regarding the issue he had heartlessly addressed.

As I continued the process over several days, I began to write about my friend instead of myself—wondering why he'd been so cruel. It dawned on me that perhaps he had been jealous of some of my accomplishments at work, and his cutting remark may have been an attempt to assert his superiority. I gained an understanding of his competitive character, and was finally able to achieve a level of acceptance and compassion. I may never fully forgive him, but I no longer harbor the malice that only makes *me* suffer more. Our relationship has changed, but we're still friends, and without the bloodletting and understanding spurred by the writing process, I might have cut off from him completely.

Writing may seem like work, but when you make the explorations I suggest in the chapters ahead, give the process a chance and you may experience the healing alchemy so well documented by Dr. Pennebaker. What explains this almost magical effect? It's hard to pinpoint, but when you entrust your deepest thoughts and feelings to a blank piece of paper or computer screen, they make no value judgments. They ask for nothing in return. If you wish, they hold your secrets forever. And if you accept their mute invitation, taking the opportunity to pour out your feelings and deepen your perceptions, you may stumble upon buried memories and unforeseen insights. Thoughts and feelings that arouse guilt may make the process harder, but if you stick with it, you gradually work them through, casting aside unnecessary and unhelpful guilt.

Affirmations and Prayer

Women can nurture spirit with affirmations that cultivate control, self-confidence, and inner peace. Chapters that follow include affirmations in the form of positive statements about one's creative potential; value as a friend, mate, or family member; health; or sexuality. You'll be encouraged to incorporate these affirmations into your daily relaxation ritual, and you'll be given space to create your own statements. During meditation, you can use simple affirmations in rhythmic concert with the ebb and flow of the breath—phrases such as "I Will/Persevere" for women with career or money troubles; "I am lovable" for women whose partners habitually criticize or belittle them; and "Still/Here" for women struggling with trauma or illness.

The healing potential of prayer is immeasurable, and you will find various prayerful statements offered in many chapters. As physician Larry Dossey showed in *Healing Words*, and as Herbert Benson demonstrated in *Timeless Healing*, the idea that prayer can aid physical healing can no longer be dismissed as magical thinking. Jeffrey S. Levin, Ph.D., Associate Professor of Family and Community Medicine at Eastern Virginia Medical School, has reviewed over 250 published empirical studies from the medical literature that show statistical relationships between spiritual practices and positive health outcomes. However, there are potential pitfalls in the way we approach prayer—for instance, out of obligation, a sense of shame, or the illusion that all our petitions will be granted as long as we are "good," moral, observant people. In chapter 9, "The Faith Factor," I describe these traps and offer you ways to evade them, while defining what I call a "self-nurturing spirituality." When pursued in a framework of self-love rather than self-negation, spiritual practice may help you to achieve tranquility, acceptance, and wisdom, if not physical health.

If you have not practiced prayer in the past, or you would like to try a simple prayerful meditation, I offer these guidelines:

• You can practice prayer exactly as you would meditation. Just choose a focus word or phrase that has a personal religious or spiritual meaning for you. The following is a list of focus words and phrases from the major religious and spiritual traditions. Don't feel constrained by this list; find the focus word or phrase that speaks to you.

Common Focus Words or Phrases for Prayer*

Christian	*Eastern*
Come, Lord	Om (the universal sound)
Lord, have mercy	*Shantih* ("Peace")
Our Father	
Our Father, who art in heaven	*Aramaic*
Lord Jesus, have mercy on me	*Marantha* ("Come, Lord")
Hail Mary	*Abba* ("Father")
The Lord is my shepherd	
Jewish	*Islamic*
Sh'ma Yisroel ("Hear, o Israel")	Allah
Echod ("One")	
Shalom ("Peace")	
Hashem ("The Name")	

*From *The Wellness Book*, Herbert Benson, M.D., & Eileen M. Stuart, R.N., M.S., Birch Lane Press, New York. 1992

Mind-Body Medicine for Self-Nurture

The methods in this chapter are basic practices; how you apply them will determine whether they enhance your creativity, relationships, self-esteem, and daily quotient of joy. Do you practice relaxation as a rigid ritual, or do you experiment with and settle on methods that speak to your deepest needs for peace of mind and self-acceptance? Do you use cognitive restructuring because I, or some therapist, suggested it, or because you recognize that challenging negative thoughts is a profoundly self-nurturing exercise? Do you write in a journal to record daily events, or do you write to work through painful emotions and free yourself from rage, despair, and self-denigration? Do you pray passively, wishing only for divine intervention to save you from stress, trauma, or self-inflicted unhappiness? Or do you pray for strength and sources of self-love that will enable you to change destructive or defeating behavior patterns?

When self-nurture guides our use of these methods for elevating mind, body, and spirit, they no longer become methods. They become extensions of our commitment to ourselves. By "ourselves," I don't mean our narrow egoistic selves, but our beautiful, worthy, expansive, compassionate selves. We must use mind-body techniques as tools to open up to ourselves and others, to find our discoverable strengths, and to recognize our goodness and deservedness from within, mining the innermost resources of mind and heart.

3

MOTHER/DAUGHTER:

NURTURING SELF IN FAMILY

A FRIEND RECENTLY told me the story of a transformative therapy session she had. Melanie had been struggling with her career and her marriage for a number of years, never seeming to move forward. She felt stuck in her job in real estate and stuck in her relationship with Jerry. I'd been hearing her concerns for years, and while I was empathetic, I did not know what it would take for her to change. While Melanie liked her therapist, she couldn't understand why she seemed to be making so little progress. One day, however, she and her therapist hit right up against the wall that had impeded her growth.

Melanie knew that intense insecurities lay at the root of her stuckness—a fear of moving on to a more challenging career and a fear of confronting Jerry with her desires for greater intimacy. But she couldn't get a handle on the causes of her shaky self-worth. In her therapy sessions, she had insisted that her parents loved her, and she couldn't fathom why or when such self-doubt had slithered into her psyche.

But during one particular session, Melanie's therapist honed in on her mother's personality. Melanie described her mother as sweet, self-effacing, and subtly depressed throughout her life. She'd been the youngest in a large family of siblings and always felt lost in the fray, unable to assert her identity with her distant parents, who were deeply involved in their hotel business. Given her history, Melanie's mother remained unassertive throughout her life, adopting the "one-down" stance in the world, which kept her from forging her own independent creative or work life.

As Melanie talked to her therapist, it was as though she were viewing her relationship with her mother through a multifaceted crystal held up to the light. But this time she was twisting it in circles, enabling her to see new shafts of illumination refracted off facets she'd never before perceived. Her old view was one-dimensional—her mother loved her and therefore her current problems must have some other cause. This session helped her recognize that her mother's love was nourishing but her mother's example was not. Melanie had unknowingly "taken in" the model her mother presented—one of a woman as a self-sacrificing people-pleaser whose deepest yearnings must remain unfulfilled. Melanie had used the fact of her relatively successful career to distinguish herself from her mother, who never had one. She now realized that she carried with her the same feelings that her mother projected: unworthiness, uncertainty, and low self-esteem.

Realizing the source of her own fragile self-worth enabled Melanie to cut through her confusion. She now saw every instance in which she gave herself short-shrift as part of her early emotional endowment, and she began to let go of her unconscious but strong identification with her mother. Melanie deepened her work in therapy, and it eventually helped her change careers and improve her marriage.

I was so struck by Melanie's story, because it illustrated how unwittingly we internalize the models our parents present to us. We internalize not only their behavior but often the emotional states they carry and communicate on subtle and not-so-subtle levels. Though it matters greatly whether our parents openly demonstrate their love and care, it also matters how they express themselves and conduct their lives. Bruno Bettelheim's simple axiom about autistic children can be applied to us all: "Love is not enough."

The capacity to self-nurture starts with our relationship with our parents, in our role as daughters. As children, did we learn the value of self-love and self-care? Did our mothers and fathers present themselves as strong models of self-nurturance, or were they ceaseless models of self-sacrifice, self-doubt, self-neglect, or even self-abuse? In our adult efforts to become more self-nurturing, do we still struggle with our parents, wrestling with phantoms of the past whenever they behave as they did when we were young? Are our current relationships with parents fraught with such issues as establishing independence, seeking unconditional love, and searching for an absent self-esteem?

Likewise, those of us who are mothers often find similar resonances in our relationships with our children, no matter what their age. Being a mother invariably raises feelings we had about our mothers and fathers, and we find ourselves unwittingly resisting or repeating their parenting behaviors with our own children. Our children's actions and emotions, setbacks and triumphs, can easily evoke our own struggles as kids, including our struggles with parents. When we are surprised by the depth of our emotional reactions with our kids—the intensity of our anger, sorrow, or love—we might look to our own familial past to uncover the origins.

The purpose of this chapter, then, is to learn how we can best nurture ourselves in our roles as daughters and mothers. My approach has two dimensions: self-nurture in solitude and in relationships. What do I mean by self-nurture in solitude? A good example is fleeing the house to take a mindful walk when our mothers push our buttons during a family visit. In contrast, an example of self-nurture in relationship is consciously choosing to spend a day with Mom in some mutually enjoyable activity, such as having lunch and catching a movie we're both dying to see. I have found that a balance between self-nurture in solitude and in relationship has a powerful long-term healing effect on ourselves as daughters and mothers.

The looming challenge as we consider our roles as daughters and mothers is simple in theory and complicated in action: How can we care for ourselves without abandoning the people we love most in the world? Carol Gilligan, the celebrated professor of education at Harvard and author of *In a Different Voice*, has sought to understand and redefine women's psychology, including, most importantly, the "feminine identification of goodness with self-sacrifice." In Gilligan's view—and mine—women have been trained throughout their lives to bestow care upon others and to leave themselves out of the universe of people who need their care.

Transformation occurs, says Gilligan, when "the woman begins to ask whether it is selfish or responsible, moral or immoral, to include her own needs within the compass of her care and concern." We should never minimize our caretaking abilities—they are among our great strengths as women. But we need to reframe our view that the only moral and responsible choices we make are those that involve taking care of others. Gilligan claims that taking care of ourselves is *also* a moral and responsible choice. In this, more than any other, realm—our relationships with parents and children—we need to internalize Gilligan's message about self-care, since our very identity depends on the sense of self we gain in these roles.

This is no easy task. But being a responsible adult often means making choices between who gets hurt in a conflict situation. Do I tell Mom I cannot visit next weekend because I have a conference I passionately want to attend? Do I miss Dad's birthday celebration in favor of a friend's baby shower? Can I inform my young daughter I cannot spend all Sunday afternoon with her because I want to take a yoga class? Gilligan does not suggest that we start inflicting small hurts on others instead of ourselves, but rather that we finally achieve balance in our relationships after a lifetime of choosing to hurt ourselves rather than risking the consequences of ever disappointing loved ones. People who say we can't please everyone all the time are wrong—we often can, if we slice ourselves into pieces. The deeper truth is that we can't please everyone if we ever hope to please ourselves, and this chapter is about protecting and caretaking ourselves in our roles as daughters and mothers.

I begin each of the following sections—body, mind, emotions, and self/spirit—emphasizing self-nurturance for ourselves as daughters, since all of us are daughters, whether or not our parents are alive. I then move to our role as mothers. Those who are not mothers may still find value in these sections, either as ways to consider future motherhood or as reflections on the mother role that may help them come to terms with their own mothers, or the images of mother they may have internalized.

Nurture the Body: Relaxing in the Mother/Daughter Role

As a Daughter

Relations with parents, past and present, can be major sources of stress in our lives, and the stress takes its toll on our bodies. *Bodies?* you might ask. Indeed. Mom calls with an intrusive question about work or marriage and the heart rate and blood pressure spikes in an instant. Dad gives us the cold shoulder when we come home for a visit and we get that nauseated feeling in the pit of our stomachs. A vacation spent with parents causes old dysfunctional dynamics to reemerge, patterns that leave us feeling powerless—and we're stuck with them for an emotionally and physically debilitating week. Even more insidiously, our parents' voices turn up in our heads during a life crisis, and if these voices are humiliating or disheartening, we end up downright depressed. Any mental health-care professional will tell you that depression is as much a phenomenon of body as of mind.

So we must nurture ourselves as daughters, and we can start in the realm of body-based relaxation. We can do so in solitude, practicing mind-body relaxation by ourselves; or we can do so in relationship, practicing relaxation when we're with parents. On occasion, we may even practice relaxation right alongside a parent as a way to overcome separateness and forge a different kind of bond.

When parents are sources of anxiety or stress, certain relaxation techniques practiced in solitude may work better than others. Though an extreme example, Marion's experience is illuminating. She grew up with a mother who, on several occasions during her early childhood, had been institutionalized for mental illness. Marion's parents were separated when she was twelve, and her father, with whom she felt safe and cared for, died when she was thirteen. Throughout her adolescence and adulthood, Marion struggled with her mother, who, without warning, could deliver a cutting remark or stinging accusation. Marion spent years in therapy working on these problems, but it wasn't until she developed a mind-body practice that she felt she could handle her mother—and her own anguish—in a healthy way.

Mindfulness meditation has been Marion's touchstone. "When I get off the phone with my mother after a difficult conversation, mindfulness gets me through," she explains. "I do my mindfulness meditation, which reorients me in the present moment. As I sit there listening to my favorite meditation tape and breathing, nothing bad is happening—my mother can't touch me. I can always find this safe place in my mind."

There are two ways you can practice mindfulness when a parent is a cause of distress, and Marion did both. Right during or after a distressing incident, you can take a step back and focus on your breathing as a trusted anchor for your awareness. Think of yourself as a mountain—solid, monumental, motionless, and changeless through time—and your mother's or father's hurtful words or actions as dark clouds passing by. Keep coming back, again and again, to your breathing and your image of yourself as a mountain. Though you may be affected—the dark clouds can shed raindrops on your terrain—you cannot be uprooted or destroyed. Your deepest self is safe in the here and now—enduring and imperturbable. You can use this approach in solitude, or even in the midst of a difficult phone call or interaction.

Another way is to practice mindfulness meditation every day as a kind of psychological "preventive medicine." Most of us carry our parents around with us through all our days and activities. Their voices, as we hear them in our minds, may be positive or negative, quiet or loud and boisterous. If we build the "muscle" of mindfulness, we will be far better able to tune out these voices when they become negative and voluble. How so? These inner tape loops are psychic remnants of the past, and a daily practice of mindfulness meditation helps relocate us in the present moment. The voices are just more dark clouds passing overhead.

Marion used other methods, as well. "I have trouble meditating when I am really depressed," she says. Many of my patients find it hard to meditate when extremely depressed, often because the effort to focus on the present is difficult—they find themselves constantly wrestling with intrusive negative thoughts. During these times, when they most need self-soothing, they quickly lose their commitment to a daily practice. Marion's solution during these times was to listen to an imagery tape of a walk on the beach. (See the appendix for the Beach Walk imagery script.) Being led by a comforting woman's voice on a pleasant seaside stroll, sensing her feet on warm sand, and viewing a vast expanse of blue ocean, Marion found respite from moments of despair.

Marion's mind-body work was not, by itself, the complete answer to all her suffering regarding her mother. Her years of therapy laid the groundwork; mindfulness meditation and imagery enabled her to till that soil, so to speak, until her sense of solidity and strength was able to flourish. Marion is convinced that she could not have made this leap forward in personal growth had she not used both psychotherapy *and* mind-body practice; in her case, the synergy was healing. There is a long and vaunted tradition of combining psychotherapy with meditation or Eastern spiritual practice, from psychoanalyst Erich Fromm in the 1950s to psychotherapist Mark Epstein in the 1990s. Marion is a case example of how therapy provides access to emotions and insights while mind-body-spirit techniques are tools that can foster serenity and personal mastery, thus allowing for a deepening of the work in therapy.

What about relaxation in relationship? I recently treated a daughter and her mother who were experiencing familial stress, in part due to the mother's cancer diagnosis. The daughter, Robin, was struggling with how to help her mother, Jean, cope with cancer treatments and decisions without becoming intrusive. This was a particular challenge for Robin, who was not convinced that Jean was choosing the best therapeutic options. Jean would blanch whenever Robin made questioning comments, even if they were subtly posed. But one approach that helped was to practice guided imagery with her mother, both during and after her radiation treatments. "I sat with her just before each radiation session, saying, 'Okay, visualize water rushing through you and see it cleaning out all the bad cells.' And, 'Focus on a bright light that's like a laser wiping out the bad stuff.' We practiced all sorts of visualizations, and it was for her benefit. But it benefited us both."

Many women have elderly parents who suffer from aches, pains, and other troubling physical symptoms. I sometimes recommend that these women teach relaxation to their parents—deep breathing, body scan, and progressive muscle relaxation, among other techniques. It brings them together, often in a profound way that heals not only the aches and pains but the tensions that can spring up, particularly between daughter and mother. (Let's face it, dads may be less likely to sit with their daughters to practice relaxation, although there will be happy exceptions.)

One of the best exercises to teach and practice with an ailing parent is autogenic training, a gentle approach with simple instructions you can read or say aloud to him or her. The script on page 41 in chapter 2 provides the phrases for use in autogenic training, and you might read them into an audiotape for your parent, who can then listen to your voice as a trusted guide through this healing relaxation technique.

As a Mother

Mini-relaxations, those short-form versions of the relaxation response (see page 42), should be to mothers what midday coffee breaks are to hard-driving careerists—essential opportunities to recharge. Certainly, every mother knows that child-rearing is the most challenging of careers. Especially during infancy, a care-taker's attention can never wane, but the juggling, scheduling, shopping, cooking, feeding, cleaning, communicating, and coordinating are endless in every phase of our children's development, through adolescence and beyond. Stress is endemic, a feature of mothers' lives as inevitable as the appearance of bad weather (unless you live in San Diego). Minis are invaluable to mothers because they can be practiced anytime, anywhere. One does not have to remove one's self from the fray in order to shift from shallow chest breathing to deep abdominal breathing, the quickest and one of the most effective stress busters in the mind-body pharmacy.

Phoebe, a thirty-five-year-old consultant who helps business employees balance work and family, has learned a few lessons of her own about self-nurture while raising her seven-year-old son, Matthew. "I use my breath to slow down and even things out," says Phoebe. She swears by mini-relaxations, which she uses on a daily basis when work and child-rearing fray her nerves. One Sunday afternoon, Matthew was helping Phoebe bake cookies, and each time she turned her back she would discover another swath of white flour on the kitchen floor. It was a perfect time for a mini-relaxation, which Phoebe would combine with a "count to 10" strategy. Instead of just breathing or just counting, Phoebe would count each abdominal breath from 1 to 10. "I'd breathe very slowly into my abdomen," she said. "It was a way to pull back and get perspective." It also eased her tensions and kept her from spiraling into anger or anxiety. Consult chapter 2 for the mini-relaxation technique that suits you best, and use it as often as you need when your child-rearing responsibilities feel overwhelming.

Remember: You don't need to walk away. The key to minis is that you can do them *in the moment.* I found this practice very useful when Sarah, at eighteen months, decided she no longer wanted to sit in the shopping cart at the grocery store. She did, however, want to grab for everything within her reach, and if I refused to buy the bag of chips that had caught her eye, she would throw a screaming fit. I live in a small town where many people know me, so Sarah's tantrums were not only upsetting but also very embarrassing. As her howls grew louder and more intense, I would remind myself to take a few deep breaths in order to regain my composure. It was reassuring to discover that as I began to feel calmer, Sarah did, too.

A good time to practice guided imagery, particularly the "distancing" kind that takes you far away to a beach, a mountain, or a meadow, is when you're feeling really overwhelmed. Your child has pushed not one but several of your most sensitive buttons and you don't know how to maintain control. In these instances, put a video on for your child and sit down on the opposite side of the room. Conscious attempts at quiet meditation may be exercises in frustration, but an imagery tape that transports you to a place of visual splendor, calming sound, or comforting memories can be a mental balm for fiery states of rage.

I also recommend a daily practice of relaxation in solitude; it can relieve chronic tensions from hard days of work or child care. This daily respite is a boon to your long-term well-being, a form of self-nurture you may need and certainly deserve. Whether you use the body scan, mindfulness, progressive muscle relaxation, meditation, or any other method, you have a right to 20 minutes each day, or even twice a day, to provide a respite to mind and body. In practical terms, this means staking your claim to that time, regardless of the circumstances. If child care is an issue, you can make your desire known to your husband, partner, or perhaps older children who can take care of younger ones. You should not pose this meekly as a request, but assertively as a fait accompli: "I am taking my time for relaxation after dinner. I'll appreciate your taking care of the baby."

Of course, there will be times when compromise is fair and appropriate. If your husband has an evening meeting and no one else is available to watch the children, you might postpone a planned session until the kids are in bed. But in general, stake your claim to time for relaxation and make it stick. Joan Borysenko, the renowned mind-body clinician, tells women to declare their intention to practice relaxation with the following demand: "I'm going into the room for 20 minutes, and I want no interruptions under any circumstance—unless it involves fire or blood."

If your children are old enough, you can teach them relaxation techniques, and even practice with them. One approach enthusiastically embraced by children and many adults is the magic-carpet guided imagery, taught to me by my late colleague Irene Goodale. Simply visualize yourself on a magic carpet, and let the carpet take you to any place of beauty or serenity that has special meaning or resonance. The magic carpet ride is a great introduction to imagery for children, since it has a Disneyesque magical quality. The image of flying can be thrilling, evoking pleasant physical sensations and a sense of limitlessness. The notion of transporting one's self to a faraway place seems both more fabulous and more possible with a magic carpet.

If your children are open to it, teach them the magic carpet imagery. Afterward, share the images and feelings that arose during the visualization. This can be a fun and instructive way to teach your children how to better manage their own stress and to nurture the body and mind when beset by negative emotions.

NURTURE THE MIND: EXITING THE PARENT TRAP

As a Daughter

The negative tape loops we learn from our parents can be the most difficult obstacles we face as we learn the art of self-nurture. That is why cognitive restructuring, the process of identifying, questioning, and ultimately changing our automatic negative thoughts from and about our parents, is the most liberating form of mind-nurture.

When I ask my patients to identify negative thoughts about their parents, or negative thoughts about themselves implanted by their parents, I get a vast variety of answers, but here are the greatest hits:

"I'm not a good enough daughter."
"Nothing I do will please Mom/Dad."
"I will never amount to anything."
"No matter how hard I try, I cannot accomplish_____."
"I can never be successful enough."
"I'm too self-centered."
"I will always undermine myself."
"I don't feel worth loving."
"I'm lazy."

Such thoughts can haunt us throughout our lives, whether our parents instilled them when we were young, or continue to do so in the present. Of course, some of us have positive tape loops as powerful or more powerful than the negative ones, thoughts that form the foundation of our self-esteem. But few of us escape childhood without being stuck with repetitive negative thoughts like those above, distorted self-assessments that rear up whenever we are challenged by life.

Reams have been written about how the daughter-mother attachment, or lack of attachment, has an overridingly powerful effect on our identities, self-worth, and capacity for self-care. Even those of us who are extremely close to our mothers can have negative tape loops just as insidious as those with distant relationships. A mother's voice of expectation, fear, or doubt is often stronger when we so desperately wish not to disappoint. As Freud once wrote, "we are never so defenseless against suffering as when we love."

Barbara, a patient who was quite close to her mother, began to discover in her forties that her attachment came with a price: a constant, nagging belief that she could never do enough to make her mother, Sandy, feel loved. While Barbara and Sandy saw each other often, Barbara felt constantly guilty because there were never enough visits, outings, and family gatherings to satisfy Sandy. Barbara used cognitive restructuring to identify her primary negative tape: "I'll never please my mother, and, therefore, I'll never feel good enough about myself."

To restructure this thought, Barbara had to break it down using the four-question method. Did the thought contribute to her stress? Surely. Where did she learn this thought? From her mother. Was it logical? The first part, about never pleasing her mother, was partially logical. Barbara certainly could please her mother, but she would never please her completely. The second part, about never feeling good enough about herself, was not logical, because it assumed that she could only feel good about herself if she completely pleased Sandy. Was the thought true? In essence, part one was true—she'd never ultimately satisfy her mother, who would not feel fulfilled no matter how much time Barbara spent with her. But part two—the truly toxic clause in Barbara's thought—was not true. Barbara did not *have to* link feeling good about herself to pleasing her mother.

Barbara's task was to disconnect her self-worth from her mother. Barbara had to recognize that she was a faithful, loving daughter, a worthwhile person who did not have to base her self-assessment on whether or not her mother was satisfied day to day, week to week, month to month. Gradually, she had to separate herself from her mother—not by pulling far away but by recognizing her own value apart from her ability to keep Sandy happy. Over time, Barbara created a new thought-structure to replace the old, damaging one: "I may never completely please my mother, but I can do a lot to please her, and I can and will feel good about myself as a daughter and a person."

I've had many patients with mothers or fathers who are overtly abusive; frequently, these parents suffer from an emotional illness. In these instances, cognitive restructuring requires us to see our parents for who they are. Melinda, forty-two, described her father as "passive" and her mother as physically and emotionally abusive. In her family system, her sister was sweet and acquiescent and her brother was perenially sick; Melinda was the one to stand up to her mother, which meant she took the brunt of the abuse. As an adult, Melinda's mother continued to make humiliating remarks, even threatening to disown her. During Christmas, she'd give presents to Melinda's siblings but none to her. While on the surface Melinda was the "strong" one in the family, she internalized the hurt and shame inflicted by her mother. "To this day, when my mother is harsh, I feel like the wicked witch at the end of *The Wizard of Oz*," says Melinda. "You know, the scene where she shrivels up and says, 'I'm melting, I'm melting.' "

In many aspects of her life, from work to family, Melinda has battled feelings of anger and shame. I was able to help by listening carefully to her descriptions of her mother's behaviors, which enabled me to confirm a borderline personality disorder. This was key to restructuring Melinda's global belief: "My mother can't stand me so I must be defective." I took out my copy of the widely used manual of psychiatric disorders, the *Diagnostic and Statistical Manual of Mental Disorders*, and read verbatim the descriptions of borderline personality disorder to Melinda. Among them were, "a pattern of unstable and intense interpersonal relationships," "recurrent suicidal threats, gestures, or behavior," and "inappropriate intense anger or lack of control of anger." I could see in her widening eyes that she recognized her mother's behavior in almost every detail. Identifying her mother's psychological disorder helped Melinda to see her in an entirely different light—not as a demon to be feared, but as a person with an illness to feel sorry for. After stating my belief that mental illnesses are biological, and as disabling as physical illnesses, I posed this question: "If your mother had cerebral palsy, would you feel so chastened and angry?"

I did not try to talk Melinda out of her feelings, or to push her into forgiving her mother. She had a right to her hurt and anger. But her continuing shame and rage, feelings that never seemed to abate, were fed by a false view of her mother, the view of the child who cannot comprehend a parent's limitations or illnesses. Melinda needed to be freed from the child's view in order to be freed from the hounding voices in her head. The restructured adult view—"My mother is emotionally ill, it's not my fault, I'm not defective"—helped her get on with her life. It even helped her to remain in touch with her mother, who was recently diagnosed with cancer. Melinda may never fully heal her relationship with her mother, but she has gone a long way toward healing her own shame and self-denigration.

Now consider the following "sample" restructurings of some of the parent-associated negative thought patterns that bedevil many women. These thoughts and restructurings may or may not directly apply to you, but they offer examples of how you can reframe punishing thoughts into ones that are kinder, gentler, and truer.

NEGATIVE THOUGHT: "I'm not a good enough daughter."

RESTRUCTURED THOUGHT: "I have tried to be a caring daughter, but my care has not always been received or appreciated."

NEGATIVE THOUGHT: "I am powerless whenever Mom/Dad is around."

RESTRUCTURED THOUGHT: "It's true that I *feel* powerless whenever Mom/Dad is around. But my sense of powerlessness has stemmed from the fact that, up till now, I've behaved as though I have no right to honestly express myself in their presence. So I'm not *actually* powerless, as long as I articulate my thoughts and assert my needs."

NEGATIVE THOUGHT: "I have no right to success."

RESTRUCTURED THOUGHT: "My parent(s) may have ingrained in me the belief that I have no right to success, but I do. I can uncover my own sense of deservedness and can learn to recognize the areas in which I *am* successful."

Practice cognitive restructuring by identifying your own negative thoughts from or about your parents, then applying the four-question approach. After you've pinpointed the thought and doggedly questioned its veracity, replace it with a thought structure that is more truthful, accurate, and kinder to yourself.

As a Mother

I'm a bad mother. This negative self-statement is certainly generic, but it is the guilt-drenched, shame-ridden belief that infects so many women and hounds their everyday sense of themselves as mothers.

If you are one of those mothers, you need to give yourself a break by practicing mind-nurture. No mother is perfect, and most of us with children would like to improve or change some of our behaviors. The desire to be a better mother is valid, but *the extent of our desire is a sign of how good we are, not how bad.* We have to stop confusing the strong wish to be the best possible mother with the conviction that we must be lousy mothers who will eventually end up in some celestial family court to answer for our misdeeds. The purpose of cognitive restructuring is not to paper over any shortcomings but to have more compassion for our limitations, to recognize when our self-criticisms are harsh and unjustified, and to become better mothers through self-awareness rather than self-punishment.

As a mother, I have had to learn these lessons repeatedly. Recently, I came home from work at 9:00 P.M. after running a group, which I do once a week, and my two-year-old daughter, Sarah, refused to acknowledge that I was home. She wouldn't even look at me, staring off into the distance while refusing to let me touch or kiss her for a good half-hour. It was the first time Sarah had ever reacted that way. I immediately criticized myself, using that old standby, "If I was a good mother, I would never work evenings." For the next half-hour, I was full of shame, and even felt abandoned by my own daughter. Then, suddenly, she turned to me and said, "Mama, pick Sarah up," and she began cuddling with me, reverting again to her normal, ebullient self.

I learned something from the experience. I recognized that my daughter was not traumatized by my absence: She was understandably upset and mad. Sarah had to find a way to express her anger, and in relatively short order she had gotten over her hurt. Had I retaliated, reacting to my own hurt by yelling or sending her to her room, her anger would surely have been exacerbated and I might have had a troubled child for hours or days. It also helped to learn from my husband that the two of them had a fine time together while I was gone. I realized that I was not harming my child by working late one evening a week, and that I did not have to let my own temporary feelings of hurt or guilt turn into an unfair assessment of myself as a mother.

In situations such as the one with my daughter, we have to ask a simple question: Am I really being neglectful, or do I just have trouble accepting that my child will sometimes, naturally, feel sad or angry when I cannot meet a particular need? Being a good mother often requires profound acceptance of the reality that we will never meet all our children's needs—an obvious point that is easily grasped by our intellects but not so by our hearts. Indeed, we are often absent because we are engaging in self-nurturing or meaningful activities that we pursue to enjoy life, exercise our creativity, or in some way become more whole. In the long run, our efforts at self-actualization mostly help our children; they make us better people and better parents.

Another everyday example comes from my friend Roxanna. She came home late from work one night and proceeded to put dinner on the table for her husband and two children: corned beef, broccoli, potatoes. Both her six-year-old daughter and eight-year-old son reviled her: "You know we hate corned beef. We're not eating this!" Some mothers would have become enraged at their children, but Roxanna's reaction was, "Oh, God, if I was a good mother I would remember that they hate corned beef." They refused to eat dinner, and Roxanna stalked into her bedroom, exhausted and tearful.

My restructuring advice to Roxanna for future incidents was to use the technique we call "Stop/Breathe/Reflect/Choose." It combines minirelaxation (deep breathing) with thought restructuring and considered action. (You literally stop, then breathe into your abdomen, then consider your choices.) To demonstrate how this might work, we did an "instant replay" of the dinner table incident. Had she stopped to reflect, she'd have realized that she was exhausted by the time she got home, having rushed to the supermarket and dashed home to get dinner on the table. Her kids were also tired, and probably frustrated that Mom had flown into the house with no time to communicate or get settled.

With reflection, she should have let herself off the hook about the corned beef, realizing that every mother makes such mistakes. And finally, rather than retreat to her bedroom, it would have made things less traumatic if she had offered a simple alternative (like a quick bowl of pasta), one in which her children would stop feeling let down and she would not have collapsed into a self-flagellating heap.

Phoebe, the mother whose young son Matthew turned their Sunday afternoon of baking cookies into an adventurous romp with white flour, was upset every time she turned around to see the mess he was making. She practiced mini-relaxations—deep breathing to calm herself so she could take a step back. But she also combined minis with cognitive restructuring. Her negative thought: "Look at this—he's making a horrible mess and I'm going to have to clean it all up." Her restructured thoughts, verbatim: "You know, we are having a really good time here. It won't take me that long to clean this up afterward. These are the moments memories are made of." Phoebe was able to laugh and let go of her anxious concerns.

Consider these cognitive restructurings of negative thoughts about yourself as a mother:

NEGATIVE THOUGHT: "I'm a bad mother because I spend too much time at work."

RESTRUCTURED THOUGHT: "I will cut back when possible, but our family needs this income and I need to realize my creative talents on the job. My children would be miserable if we were financially insecure and I was chronically dissatisfied. I'm quick to label myself as 'bad' because I am not mothering the way my mother did. But I live in a different time, and when I look at the whole picture, I realize that I am a good mother."

NEGATIVE THOUGHT: "My child's poor performance at school is my fault."

RESTRUCTURED THOUGHT: "I am not responsible for everything my children do. Many factors, including social and genetic ones, are totally

beyond my control. I'm doing the best I
can to help him/her with school work,
and I can only encourage him/her to do
the best he/she can."

NEGATIVE THOUGHT: "My children never appreciate all that I do
for them."

RESTRUCTURED THOUGHT: "I must do the best I can and then have
faith, knowing that my love and support
is intrinsically nourishing for my
children, and that I will come to feel
worthy as a mother, no matter how
much they do not express or show it."

Use these examples as templates to help you identify your own negative thought patterns about yourself as a mother, and to develop more
truthful and compassionate restructured thoughts.

NURTURE THE EMOTIONS:
BEYOND GRIEF AND ANGER

As a Daughter

A woman with solid self-esteem has most likely been blessed by parents
who, during childhood, were available, caring, and capable of unconditional love. Yet many of us were wounded as daughters, and the foundations of our self-esteem were thus weakened. We may be aware of these
wounds, or we may not. We may identify too strongly with our wounds,
going through life feeling perpetually defensive or furious, or we may
deny the existence of any such wounds. Frequently, whether or not we
realize it, we try to get others to salve our wounds—loved ones, children,
friends, employers, or the very parents who inflicted those wounds in
the first place.

The people close to us in our lives can sometimes help us to heal
hurts of the past caused by insensitive or abusive parents, whose mis-
treatment was often unwitting. But ultimately, there is no one other
than ourselves who can initiate and complete the process of emotional
healing. The struggle to get others to fulfill unmet needs from the past,
or to compensate for old pains, can be a sources of trouble—a direct
contributor to chronic desperation, obsessive relationships, ongoing

conflicts with husbands and children, even divorce. No matter how loving, people in our present cannot be the parents we wish we'd had. For women who've been wounded, emotional self-nurture involves turning within for the strength to acknowledge and accept our losses; grieve for past wounds; offer ourselves the loving care we have missed; and ask significant others not to heal our hurts but to stand with us as we heal ourselves.

As with nurturing the body, in which I teach relaxation in solitude and relationship, nurturing emotions involves *awareness in solitude* and *expression in relationship*. Emotional awareness in solitude—becoming conscious of feelings that drive everyday thoughts and behaviors—can be brought about in many ways. Certainly, a skilled psychotherapist can help us become aware of repressed emotions or memories that form the basis for many of our current behavior patterns and chronic problems. Counseling and therapy is often the best way to work through these feelings and issues, and I recommend psychotherapeutic treatment for all women who are wounded in ways that damage their relationships or quash their potential for lives of purpose and meaning. But, as we will shortly see, it is also possible to sharpen emotional awareness through exploratory writing, and it is possible to effectively express emotions about our parents—or to them—by honing our communication skills.

Awareness and expression of emotions regarding our parents is the fundamental form of emotional self-nurture, for reasons that are largely accepted by most psychologists and therapists. These reasons are nicely summarized by Maggie Scarf in her illuminating book *Intimate Worlds: Life Inside the Family*:

> We take this first environment of our lives inside us as a rough-hewn interior blueprint for later emotional relating. The nurturing, enculturating family is the place in which we learn about what kinds of feelings are acceptable, appropriate, and tolerable—and what feelings are not allowable at all. As Dr. Theodore Lidz points out in *The Person*, "It is in the family that patterns of emotional reactivity develop and interpersonal relationships are established that pattern and color all subsequent relationships."

Thus, a first step toward emotional awareness in solitude is to reveal to ourselves that "rough-hewn interior blueprint for emotional relating." How did our basic orientation to all other relationships begin in our relations with our mother and father? Were there early wounds that still influence our behavior and ways of relating? Do early patterns and emotions determine whether we fear or crave intimacy with men? With other women? In the present, do we feel loved by our parents? (If one or both are not alive, do we carry with us a sense of their love and care?) The more completely we bring to the surface and understand these complex webs of feeling, the more fully we honor our emotional selves—my definition of emotional self-nurture.

You can begin with a series of simple writing explorations about your parent(s) to help you develop emotional awareness in solitude as discussed in chapter 2. The first writing exercise is offered to help you open up regarding your relationship with one or both of your parents:

> **1. Ask yourself if you are dissatisfied with your relationship with one or both of your parents. For now, pick the one with whom you feel most dissatisfaction. (If one or both parents are deceased, select a parent with whom you felt dissatisfaction.)**
>
> **Now, write your deepest thoughts and feelings about whether and how you feel loved by this parent. Do you feel unloved, or unhappy with the way they express their love? Is their love conditional or constraining? Write about your frustration, sadness, anger, and situations that have evoked those emotions. Let the feelings flow in an unimpeded fashion. As you continue the process over several sessions, see if you can understand more about your feelings and behavior, as well as their feelings and behavior.**

Psychologist James Pennebaker, a leading researcher in writing explorations, reports that some people practicing his technique can't think of any major trauma or stressful circumstance. That's okay. Instead, they begin writing about small irritations, the everyday hassles to which none of us are immune, and gradually, these details lead inexorably to some previously unacknowledged grief or anger, even to memories long unexplored. Many women in my groups who practice the writing exercise have had this experience. One of my infertility patients, Paula, wrote about her distress over the rigors of fertility treatment and the marital strain she continued to endure. This alone was helpful, but soon Paula realized that her anguish was intensified by her belief that she had no right to be a mother, that she somehow deserved her infertile fate.

As she wrote out her pain, Paula traced her merciless inner judgment to an abortion she had had a decade earlier. Paula had unconsciously harbored shame about the abortion throughout her three-year struggle with infertility. By her second day of writing, Paula traced this guilt to her parents, who had been unwaveringly strict in their religious training. She could only imagine their outrage had they learned of her abortion. Of course, she hid the abortion from her mother and father, but she could not hide from the parents she'd internalized. Paula never overcame her guilt about the abortion, and she saw her inability to give birth as a form of parental or divine punishment—or both.

By the third day, Paula used the writing exploration to confront the psychic baggage from her parents—to realize just how merciless she'd been toward herself. On the third and fourth day of writing, she began to lift the weight of shame from her shoulders. Paula's self-forgiveness was healing, but might never have occurred had she not first recognized and processed her guilt. I've had countless other patients with a variety of disorders, from infertility to PMS to depression, recognize similarly burdensome psychological issues linked to their parents that either caused or worsened their suffering.

Consider this sample of one woman's writing exercise, showing the progression of emotions and insights over the course of several days. Here is a brief excerpt from Randy's first day of writing, a memory of an event that occurred when she was six:

> My father couldn't stop slamming the door. He was screaming at my mother and slamming the bedroom door over and over. I kept yelling, "Daddy stop it, stop it, please!" Finally, he turned to me and said, "Get in your room and shut the door." I started to cry and he just yelled louder at me to go to my room. I couldn't comprehend that he would not react to my crying, that my crying made no difference. It didn't stop him, it didn't make him worry about me. I was so hurt and frightened. He was like a machine. I think from that day on I never completely trusted him again.

Here is an excerpt from Randy's writing on day three:

> I know my mom and dad had major problems around finances. She was always buying stuff and he was always trying to rein her

in. I can see his point of view about all this now. He wasn't the only one who could be difficult; she was no day at the beach. He was always worried about money and she had some kind of serious shopping addiction. I think he was just out of control that day when I tried to stop him from screaming at her. At that moment I lost some trust in him, and that will always sadden me. But this has made me scan my brain for a more complete picture. Was he really that bad? I can remember good moments, like the time I came home with a pretty crummy report card and he sat me down and told me not to worry, that he knew I'd do better, that I should be proud of myself.

Note the raw emotion Randy experienced on day one, the undisguised anguish she articulated with such clarity. By day three, Randy had a different perspective and new insights. Having confronted her most upsetting and disillusioning moment with her father, she was then able to move toward a more penetrating and compassionate perspective on him as both a husband and father.

Self-Nurture and Anger: A Healing Connection

The most vexing emotion for many daughters is—big surprise—anger. But you may ask, what does anger have to do with self-nurture? Everything—because healthy expression of anger is synonymous with assertiveness, the ability to stand up for yourself in relations with parents, children, friends, employers, or anyone who has some power over you. We cannot be genuinely self-nurturing if we cannot be assertive. Self-nurture is about much more than treating ourselves to a nice movie or pleasant massage once in a while. It is about reclaiming our right to pleasure and wholeness, and it requires us to make strong statements to loved ones about our limits, boundaries, and needs.

Our self-protective capacity for assertiveness clearly stems, in large part, from our early relations with our parents. Most of us were brought up not to express anger toward our parents, which is why we have so much deflected or compacted fury embedded in our psyches. Suppressed anger can produce a variety of ill effects. With regard to relationships, those of us who consciously suppress or unconsciously repress anger often end up being mistreated, since we don't have anger in our emotional repertoire to defend ourselves. We tend toward passivity, masochism, or passive-aggressive "acting out," all of which erode the quality of our relationships, making it immensely difficult to get our needs met, to be known by loved ones for our authentic selves. On the physical side, those of us who perenially quash anger become susceptible to headaches, back pain, gastrointestinal diseases, and, according to some research, serious disorders of the immune system.

Some women at the other extreme are compulsive expressers, venting fury at the flimsiest provocation. As Harriet Goldhor Lerner characterized so clearly in *The Dance of Anger*, explosively angry women are no better off than amicable repressors. When we "dump" rather than communicate anger in a clean, nonblaming manner, we alienate those we love and risk the deterioration of relationships that, in our hearts, we wish to strengthen rather than undermine. Lerner points out that anger is an alarm bell, a signal that something is wrong in our relationships or ourselves. The best way to express anger is the manner that most effectively redresses unfairness or gets our needs met. For instance, if we feel that our father is treating us with disdain, screaming at him is not likely to elicit the response we want. But if we calmly and respectfully let him know that his insults sting and that we only wish for more understanding and affection from him, we may achieve our underlying goal. Assertiveness as opposed to rageful outbursts is usually the most effective way to communicate anger.

To make this transformation, we must first come to terms with how *we* handle anger. Did our parents or other caregivers frustrate our basic emotional needs, giving us continual cause to be angry? Did they allow us to express anger in appropriate ways? How did *they* express it? Did they model healthy assertiveness, or one of the unhealthy extremes—passivity or aggressiveness?

You might explore your relationship to anger vis-à-vis your parents in the following writing exploration:

2. Write your deepest thoughts and feelings about the time in your past when you were most angry at your parents. Write both facts—what happened, how you reacted or did not react—and feelings—the quality of the anger you felt inside, whether or not you openly expressed it during the event.

This exercise will put you directly in touch with intensely emotional memories and insights about your relationships with parents. The following exercise focuses on your parents as models for your own emotional expression. It should help you understand your own style of emotional expression:

3. Write about each of your parents and their way of expressing themselves. How did they each relate to anger? Were they passive, never expressing anger? Or did they explode in fury whenever something went wrong? Alternatively, did they communicate angry feelings in a balanced, nonblaming manner? What might you have learned from your parents as models of how to manage anger?

These exercises will give you a sure grasp of the nature and origins of your own style of managing and expressing anger. Now the question arises, How can I express anger more effectively? While the writing explorations should ground you in self-understanding, it's important for you to evaluate how your past has influenced your present. Ask yourself: Can I manage anger more effectively today with my parents? Other family members? Children? Coworkers? Friends? People who remind me of my parents?

To effect change in how you manage anger, it helps to have clear guidelines for healthy means of expression. A worthy goal is to develop your ability to be assertive, as opposed to aggressive, passive, or passive-aggressive. Assertiveness is the controlled use of anger, not to punish people we feel have done us wrong, but to get our needs met. In our Division of Behavioral Medicine, we teach assertive communication skills using the following simple quadrant:

ASSERTIVE	**AGGRESSIVE**
Communication Reflects:	Communication Reflects:
I count.	I count.
You count.	You don't count.
PASSIVE-AGGRESSIVE	**PASSIVE**
Communication Reflects:	Communication Reflects:
I count.	I don't count.
You don't count, but I'm not going to tell you this.	You count.

Your first surge of anger is often aggressive in quality, and acting on that surge without reflection can be dangerous—the "I count, you don't count" message that is off-putting at best and inflammatory at worst. Once in a blue moon, acting on such impulses is self-protective. If you are physically assaulted on the street, it would not be particularly useful to say, "I'm upset by your behavior and truly wish you'd find another way to channel your rage." You'd probably be better off screaming, "Get off me or I'll call the cops!" When your child has undergone surgery and her doctor refuses to give her enough pain medication, and your assertive comments have failed, you have every reason to raise your voice. (Actress Shirley MacLaine demonstrates clean, aggressive anger in the film *Terms of Endearment.* When a nurse refuses to administer pain medication to her dying daughter, played by Debra Winger, MacLaine's character has an unforgettable, uninhibited hissy fit on the hospital ward. Suddenly the nurse can't get the pills fast enough.)

But these are relative exceptions. Most often, it's in your best interest to follow the "Stop/Breathe/Reflect/Choose" guideline. This approach enables you to consider the most effective, assertive words and actions possible. The question is, Can we lose our tempers in a controlled manner that clearly communicates our feelings and goals? Yes, if we choose words and behaviors that help us meet the specific need that has been frustrated. Our anger should be used to rectify the imbalance or injustice that set off the alarm bells in the first place, not to vent with hurtful generalizations.

This rule of thumb is especially important in dealing with our parents in the present. Consider this example: Your mother tells you she has other plans and therefore will not come to the gallery opening of your new show of paintings. You feel hurt that she doesn't seem to care about something very important to you. You want her, at least, to acknowledge how upset you are. Now choose between these two divergent ways of expressing your severely bruised feelings. You scream, "You never support my work!" and call her "selfish," or "uncaring." Or, you sit down at the kitchen table and articulate your disappointment: "I wanted you to come and my feelings were hurt when you said you wouldn't. I want to feel that you care about my creative work, which is one of the most important parts of my life." Which approach is more likely to rectify what hurt you in the first place and serve in the future to improve understanding between you and your mother? Which might prompt her to change her plans, or at least set the stage for a different outcome next time you have a gallery show?

Passivity is perhaps the least self-nurturing choice as an ongoing strategy for managing anger, one that is rarely consciously chosen but that we gradually adopt as a psychological path of least resistance. Passive aggression is no better, a sneaky way of acting out anger without taking responsibility for it. Those of us who rely on passive aggression don't acknowledge or express anger; we bottle it up while remaining passive on the surface. But that doesn't prevent our anger from leaking out in insidious ways, small acts of martyrdom or covert punishments of people with whom we have a grievance.

A close friend recently told me the story of her anniversary celebration with her husband, who had neglected to give her flowers or a gift. When she and her husband went out for a celebratory dinner, my friend proceeded to critique his choice of restaurants, nitpick over his manners ("Will you ever learn how to hold a fork and knife?"), and dredge up decades-old gripes. She never said, "I'm hurt that you did not give me flowers or a gift." Had she, a brief chat and heartfelt apology would have prevented the evening from spiraling into a psychic fencing match. She had fallen back on a classic form of passive aggression, which is virtually always self-defeating.

Assertiveness is the healthy path because it implies that "I count and you count." "I count" because I take the difficult and often courageous chance of stepping forth with my true emotions, as troubled or unpleasant as they may be. And "you" (the other) count because I step forth respectfully, taking care not to use aggressive tactics of bullying or blame. Rather, I focus on *my* feelings, not *your* faults; I state my hurt, disappointment, or anger, and I make clear my desire to be heard and understood. My goal should not be to exact vengeance, but to restore a sense of fairness (especially in work relationships or dealings with people in public) or to reestablish intimacy (especially in close friendships or family relationships).

At the same time, managing anger through assertiveness is not the only form of emotional self-nurture for daughters. Developing communication skills with parents is a multifaceted task—clarifying needs and wishes, avoiding traps of dependency or disconnectedness, maintaining psychological balance in the face of disapproval or anxiety, knowing when to exercise control and when to relinquish it.

Earlier I told you about Robin, the woman who struggled with how to help her mother, Jean, who was undergoing treatment for breast cancer. Robin and her sister did not agree with the manner in which Jean and their father, Martin, were handling her cancer crisis. Robin felt they should research options, get second opinions, query their doctors. Instead, they were accepting their oncologist's treatment plan without question. Robin was having increasingly unpleasant conversations with Jean and Martin, trying to force them to see her point of view and to reorient their approach. Robin believed she was trying to save her mother's life; Jean felt she was pursuing the best treatment prescribed by a doctor in whom she'd placed her trust.

While I validated Robin's emotional state, I gently challenged her strategy. I pointed out that her parents were part of a generation that did not question doctors. "True, my sister and I are from the Watergate era," said Robin. "We question everybody." Robin began to realize that her and her sister's efforts to gain control over Jean's cancer treatment decisions were upsetting every member of the family, causing more strife at a time when Jean needed less strife in her support system. "I had to understand that my parents were their own people. The fact that my mother was unassertive made me want to seize control and care for her. I had to be reminded that she had her own way of going about this process, and I had to respect that."

But this was not an easy task. Robin came to me saying that her parents' passive approach was a source of real distress, fueling her impulse to direct her mother's health-care decision-making. I told Robin not to judge her own emotional responses. Instead, I suggested that she write them out in a journal. Explore every shadow and shade of anxiety, anger, and bewilderment, I said. Let it all out on paper, and you won't have to let it out on them.

Robin took my advice. "I wrote out all my feelings about my mother's illness and my frustrations with my parents' way of doing things. I don't know if I kept this journal consistently enough, or whether I did it well. But I know it helped. It allowed me to have my feelings and to validate them for myself."

In her journal, it was okay to be aggravated with her parents' passive approach. Robin's feelings, and even her wish to control, were not crazy; they were understandable. But it was not wise for her to act on all those feelings. Her increasingly unhappy experiences with her parents were proof that trying to wrest control was counterproductive. Letting go of her frustrations in her journal helped Robin let go of her desire to control Jean and Martin.

The more Robin let go of her desire for control, the more compassion she had for her parents—and for herself. "In my journal, one thing always came back," she recalls. "That was to take it easy on myself."

Robin's writing explorations enabled her to make an essential shift. She began asking fewer questions of her parents and changed her approach from challenging to respectful. She no longer insisted on joining Jean at doctor's appointments, or learning every new detail of her treatment plan. Robin surrendered control, but she also struck a fine balance, refusing to distance herself from her mother's struggle. When she did have questions, she'd phrase them delicately, mentioning her concerns with compassion and a light touch.

Jean lived for several years after her cancer diagnosis. No longer engaged in a tug-of-war over medical issues, Robin and her mother were able to enjoy each other's company. Robin saw a profound change in Jean, who was clearly heartened that the tension between them had finally subsided. Struggle gave way to a new depth of communication, though it was tinged with the sorrowful recognition that Jean's time was limited. Robin did not see Jean's impending death as a sign of her failure to intervene, or Jean's failure to follow her advice. Robin had put that thinking behind her, recognizing that she could not have guaranteed her mother's survival, and that surrendering control had brought her something precious she never expected: a healing of their relationship.

Robin later told me that her writing "forced me to find the precise word that really describes what you are feeling." The practice led her back to an old interest in poetry, and after Jean died, Robin wrote a poem for her memorial service. "I had learned how to free associate, so after my mother died, I threw down all sorts of words that came to mind," she said. "Then I began to focus on words, very specific words, that captured and clarified how I felt about my mother." It was only fitting that the writing process, which brought such needed change to their relationship, also gave Robin the "voice" to create such a loving tribute to her mother.

As a Mother

If you are a mother, you can initiate emotional self-nurture by identifying aspects of yourself as a mother that cause stress or anguish. Are you so harried by daily responsibilities that your need to set priorities leaves you wondering whether you've slighted your children? Or do you fear that you won't properly meet your child's every need, no matter how relatively minor, and thus find yourself perpetually awash in guilt? Are you a mother with a short fuse, who frets after every scream session that you might have mistreated your child? Or are you the kind of mother so averse to the merest display of anger that you bend over backwards to be accommodating, even when a child needs clear limit-setting? Are you the kind of mother who *invariably* gives short shrift to your own self-nurturing needs in favor of your child, even when other caretakers are available to take up the slack?

I see mothers who err on one side or the other of these multiple equations; in most instances, the healthy middle ground is repeatedly missed. Here is a quick review of these mothering styles with succinct recommendations for emotionally self-nurturing correctives.

The Harried Mother: The harried mom is frequently overwhelmed by child-care and work responsibilities. Her anger is an outgrowth of stress and a short fuse, and her guilt stems from the feeling that she has too little of that precious commodity—"quality time"—with children whose needs are often experienced as burdensome. She may set limits too rigidly, either because she follows the parenting model from her family of origin, or because she feels she has too little time, energy, or focus to work through difficult emotional or practical problems with her kids. She is often the working mom, the single mom, or the financially stretched mom, whose daily schedule is as crammed as a crayon box and who is daunted by the seemingly impossible task of meeting her family's needs and her own.

Emotional self-nurture for the harried mom includes:

1. Taking time alone for quiet reflection, meditation, and pleasurable activities. Harried mothers may have the least time available for such "nonproductive" pursuits, but they also need this respite more than most. Body-based relaxations that

emphasize the breath (breath focus, body scan) and release of muscular tensions (progressive muscle relaxation) are especially useful. Harried mothers tell me how surprised they are by the refreshing payoff from 20 minutes of dedicated relaxation—it often yields hours of renewed energy.

2. Actively pursuing "down time" with children that has nothing to do with schoolwork or meals. That means quiet time to talk or engage in purely fun activities—playing board games, reading stories, joining them in outdoor sports—that reawaken you to the joys of motherhood. Otherwise, it's all car pools, lunch boxes, and haggling over homework.

3. Writing to explore daily events that trigger your anger. Specifically, write your deepest thoughts and feeling about events in which your child pushed your buttons. You may uncover past traumas, or current-day stressors that have nothing to do with your child, which make you vulnerable to an inappropriate or explosive response. All mothers are susceptible—you've had it up to here with your job, or your husband has been no help around the house, and a garden-variety issue with your kid turns into a full-blown row. Use writing as both a diagnostic—to find the underlying source of trouble—and as a steam-valve release. If writing doesn't help you resolve such ongoing incidents, you may need the on-going help of a therapist to help you manage anger with your child in a healthier fashion.

The Shame-Based Mother: The shame-based mother has internalized a noble concept of mothering rooted in an irrefutable truth: My child's needs come first. But taken to an extreme, this noble concept ceases to serve either the child's or the mother's deepest needs adequately. Children's needs do come first, but if mother's needs are perpetually sacrificed, the balance shifts so completely that children become saddled with more power than they need or can handle. The shame-based mother always feels she's not doing enough; she worries that her child's everyday struggles could be traumatic, leading her to intervene anxiously at every turn to make everything okay. Often, such mothers were not well nurtured by their mothers, and they've made an unconscious vow to compensate for their losses by never missing an opportunity to nurture their own children. The shame-based mother finds herself exhausted and ultimately frustrated for two reasons. First, she never feels she can do enough for her child, and she's saddled with guilt over her perceived shortcomings. Second, her child may eventually develop difficulties with separation and individuation—becoming his own person in the world who recognizes his own capacity for nurturing himself.

Emotional self-nurture for the shame-based mother includes these steps:

1. Gradually release yourself from the grip of guilt over not providing ceaseless nurturance; that means letting your child find her own solutions to some problems without interjecting your care at every step. For instance, the next time your children fight with each other, don't instantly intervene. See if they can figure out their own solution.
2. Let yourself off the hook by having compassion for yourself as a mother who, like almost all mothers, is imperfect but trying her best. Know that your style and beliefs are an understandable outgrowth of your own upbringing. No additional shame over feeling shame! As your goal, replace "perfect mothering" with "good-enough mothering."
3. Grant yourself full permission for time to enjoy purely relaxing and/or pleasurable activities.
4. Write about your feelings of anxiety and shame to relieve pressure and to forge deeper insights about the origins of your mothering style.

The Self-Denying Mother: Harried mothers, shame-based mothers, and many others are also, typically, self-denying mothers. The self-denying mother is relentlessly angry or guilty or worried about her children. All mothers must sacrifice certain needs in order to be responsible, loving parents. But the self-denying mother loses her balance in applying this principle. She goes overboard in sacrificing self, often because she's driven by obligation and shame to please everyone else before she pleases herself.

The self-denying mother must cultivate an unwavering commitment to self-nurture—of body, mind, emotions, and spirit. In my effort to motivate such mothers to make this commitment, I ask two simple questions: By endlessly giving and doing, are you depleting yourself? When you are physically and spiritually exhausted, are you the best mother you can be? The answer to the former is always yes, and the answer to the latter is always no. When these mothers contemplate their answers, they're usually ready to make the leap toward self-nurture.

The self-denying mother must be wise and flexible as she searches for and grasps blocks of time to tend to herself. She must also be willing to procure all the help she needs from her partner and other caretakers. At the same time, she must give herself time to change, for the guilt she feels when she puts herself first is very deeply ingrained. Indeed, she typically has transformed that guilt into an entrenched child-rearing style or philosophy in which her needs always take a back seat. The self-denying mother must be willing to modify her child-rearing approach to better serve herself and her kids.

A good example is my friend Jennifer, a self-denying mother who is genuinely devoted to her three children. But Jennifer has trouble setting limits, so she spends inordinate amounts of time offering her children infinite choices. Once when I was visiting Jennifer, we decided to go out with her kids for a treat. I waited for a full fifteen minutes in her driveway, standing there speechless as she consulted her nine-year-old daughter regarding choices of ice-cream parlors. They ran down every 7-Eleven, Friendly's, and other favored joints in the neighborhood. Finally, Jennifer's daughter made her selection. For years, Jennifer has complained that she has no time for herself, that she feels emotionally and physically overwhelmed. No wonder! In my mind, I multiplied that fifteen minutes by the number of times such a scenario probably played out in her private daily life with her children, and I was surprised Jennifer found time to eat and sleep.

Harried, shame-based, and self-denying mothers can all stand to learn the lessons of assertiveness. The harried mom tends toward aggressiveness with her children, the shame-based mom is passive, and self-denying moms can be aggressive, passive, and, quite often, passive-aggressive. Mothers do well to view their responses to daily events through this lens: Am I reacting with aggression, passivity, passive aggression, or assertiveness? Let the quadrant on page 78 be your guide. If you pay careful attention, you'll find a dozen challenges every day for which you can choose the path of assertiveness. For instance, your fourteen-year-old daughter wants you to organize her birthday party, and you're delighted to do so. But she unceremoniously drops this bombshell: "I want it to be a coed slumber party." What do you do? The passive response: "Well, sure, okay, I'm not thrilled but I'll help," you say, your voice trailing off into a stupified whisper. The aggressive response: "Of course you can't have a coed slumber party! Do you think this house is a bordello?" you scream. The passive-aggressive response: "Okay, whatever, have your party," you snort. But when party time comes, you are the soul of inhospitality, sniping at your daughter and her friends. The assertive response: "I think you're too young to have a co-ed party, so you have a choice: Have your female friends over for a slumber party, or have a co-ed dinner but not a sleepover," you say in a firm, calm tone of voice.

Being assertive with your children is supremely self-nurturing, because it demonstrates mutual respect, draws clear-cut boundaries, and makes space for both your children's needs and your own. Self-nurture must be negotiated in such a way that you don't inflict gratuitous pain on the people you love, especially your children.

NURTURE THE SELF/SPIRIT: SEPARATE, SATISFIED, SERENE

As a Daughter

Melinda, the woman whose mother suffered from a personality disorder, used cognitive restructuring to realize, "My mother is emotionally ill, it's not my fault, I'm not defective." She paid a price for being the one member of her family to be assertive with her mother, shouldering her abuse throughout her childhood, adolescence, and adulthood. In Melinda's view, she and her siblings experienced the kind of familial anguish that left each of them unable or unwilling to start families of their own. "My sister is forty-four, my brother is forty-one, and I am forty-two, and none of us has children," she said forlornly. "I bet that has not evolved by accident. I married an older man who I felt certain would not put pressure on me to have children. My sister married an older man who already has children. We make choices for reasons; I just felt that children would be too painful."

In her sessions with me, Melinda worked with commitment and courage to nurture body, mind, emotions, self, and spirit. She let herself off the hook with regard to her mother's abuse, regularly practiced relaxation, reframed her view of her mother as sick rather than malevolent, and expressed her anger and shame in the safe context of therapy. I also encouraged her to treat herself with a merciful tenderness, making time for pleasurable activities—massages, yoga classes, special dates with her husband, solo outings to movies or galleries.

After this crash course in self-nurture, Melinda's feelings about having children changed. Taking such good care of herself had a healing effect on the daughter within and, hence, on the prospective mother within. Freeing herself from the albatross of her internalized image of defective "mother," and fully coming into her own as a woman and a person, Melinda began to imagine herself as a loving mother with an emotionally and physically healthy child.

"I had spent forty-one years of my life fearing I would be like my mother, and preferring not to have children than to be like her," Melinda told me in a recent conversation. "But I changed a lot in my work with you. I remember you once saying to me, 'Can you think of being a mother as your opportunity to do it better, to do it right?' I now feel that I could do a really good job at it, and I had never felt that way." Given her age, Melinda is having to seek fertility treatment in her efforts to become pregnant, but she is optimistic about her chances.

Such is the power of nurturing self and spirit to help us move forward in our lives. Not only was Melinda's dark view of motherhood altered, her whole worldview was transformed.

To nurture self and spirit as a daughter, consider using these positive affirmations—statements to repeat inwardly to yourself in meditation or in the midst of stressful encounters or ongoing conflicts with your parents. Use the affirmations that best fit your relationship with a parent or the particulars of a present problem:

> You gave me life, but I don't owe you my life.
> I deserve to care for myself.
> I have a right to your unconditional respect and care.
> I won't live to prove myself to you.
> It's never going to be perfect.
> Separate, satisfied, serene.
> I don't have to live out your unfulfilled dreams.
> I am nourished by your love, despite your limitations.

These affirmations can liberate you from the self-negating constraints that your parents have imposed or that you've internalized in your psyche.

Part of nurturing self and spirit vis-à-vis parents is to reframe your expectations of them. If your expectations are too high, you may want more than they can give, which will make it difficult for you to separate from them. Healthy separation, a process frequently derailed in adolescence when it would normally occur, requires that we accept our parents' shortcomings and move on to find full acceptance from others and ourselves. But healthy separation requires us to integrate the sadness of losing the mother or father of our fantasies. Many adult women retain illusions about their parents, illusions that keep them struggling to get the unconditional love they missed and that continues to elude them. That struggle can become the source of a prolonged agony, since the "goods" are never forthcoming. It is far better for daughters to let go of their illusions about their parents, even though this inevitably means feeling the sadness of *disillusionment*. Disillusionment sounds depressing, but in this context it is transformative; shedding our illusions about parents ends our fruitless struggles to change them, allowing us to relate to them as autonomous people. Disillusionment also prompts us to turn to ourselves, our significant others, children, and friends to meet needs our parents cannot.

If your expectations of parents are too high, you can use affirmations to let go of your illusions. Consider using these positive statements in conjunction with prayer or meditation: "I won't live to prove myself to you," "It's never going to be perfect," "Separate, satisfied, serene."

Such statements are both sad and liberating. When you surrender false images of your parents ("It's never going to be perfect"), you embrace the sorrow that is inevitable in almost every parent/child relationship. But this sorrow is also a prerequisite for becoming a separate person capable of emotional and spiritual self-nurture. After years or decades, you can finally relieve yourself of impossible expectations that keep you locked in anguish about the perfect mother or father you never had.

But what if your expectations are too low? This is common among daughters whose parents are so distant or conditional in their affection that relating to them seems like a painful chore. Such daughters often detach, defending themselves from potential hurt by expecting little and asking for less. But the pain persists, and such daughters may do well to confront their mothers or fathers, using the assertiveness and communication skills described above. For these daughters, spiritually affirming statements include, "I have a right to your respect and care," and "It's never going to be perfect."

Daughters with parents who are "toxic"—physically or verbally abusive—must often separate completely, or confront such parents with absolutely firm boundary-setting behaviors. For these daughters, affirmations include, "I don't have to live out your legacy," "I don't owe my life to you," "I deserve to care for myself."

Many daughters find themselves trapped in the role of caretaking for their mothers, providing bottomless quantities of emotional help and practical support. We all know when listening is no longer an offering but an obligation, when giving support is an exhausting drag rather than an act of openheartedness in a two-way street. Such imbalanced mother-daughter relations require us to step back, recognize the pattern, and take the self-nurturing step of saying no when necessary or desirable.

A friend, Ruth, recently described her relationship with her mother in vivid terms: "When we talk, it's like I hear this great sucking sound. At the end of a conversation, I feel I have nothing left." Ruth asked for my advice, and I told her that she's halfway home—many women in one-way relationships with their parents don't even recognize how depleted they become. I suggested that she begin limiting the overlong, unilateral conversations by openly explaining that she's tired. Ruth shot back, "I do that!" To which I asked, "After how long?" "Over an hour." I told her that seemed awfully long, and that she should give herself a half-hour limit. Beyond this time management, I also suggested that she begin asking her mother to listen more to *her* problems. Ruth said, "I'm not sure I *want* to tell her my problems."

I've heard Ruth's response from many women. I pressed her on this point: "If you don't want to share *anything* about your life, that suggests that you don't really want much of a relationship." She agreed, deciding that in truth she *did* want to talk to her mother, at least about certain facets of her life. We talked about how Ruth could assertively communicate that she wished her mother would ask about her life and be willing to listen more. Her mother was taken aback at first, but she was ultimately responsive, recognizing that Ruth's motive was to create a closer, more authentic relationship between them. We must clue our mothers in to our limits and our desires, using language that is both assertive and compassionate.

For daughters with parents who require caretaking due to an illness or infirmity, setting limits may be harder. But you can and must, either by taking breaks, hiring more help if you can afford to, and assertively procuring other family members (siblings, aunts, uncles), friends, and neighbors to assist you. The literature on the psychological and physical ill-effects associated with the stress of caretaking sick and/or elderly parents is growing exponentially. Don't wait until *you* are sick to get the help you need to be a sane, healthy, and effective caretaker. The best affirmations for caretaker-daughters are "I'm doing the best I can" and "I deserve to care for myself."

Beyond affirmations, you can nurture self/spirit by spending quality time with parents doing things you both enjoy. This requires some creativity, since we normally lapse into family activities of a stultifying sameness—the holiday turkey dinner, the perennial summer retreat, the evening party at our least favorite uncle's, and so forth. Try suggesting to your mother that you attend a lecture together on a subject—say, literature, movies, alternative medicine—or anything you're both passionate about. If your interactions with your mother are always embedded in the family system, with all its repetitive dynamics, make a special effort to spend time alone with her at lunch, the theatre, or a bookstore.

Try to engage your father in a setting that changes the emotional temperature between you. If you recall some activity you enjoyed as a child with him (long walks on neighborhood streets, country drives, fly fishing), suggest that you do one of them. You might rekindle the sense of ease of being with your father, or settle into an ease you never had before.

If you share a religious affiliation or practice with your parents, you might accompany them to a church, mosque, or synagogue. A daughter's spiritual self-nurture has many shades, among them private affirmations and prayers. But you might also share your spiritual journey with your parents. If you're comfortable doing so, joining them in prayer can yield the peace of mind that comes with seeing yourselves as individuals and as a family unit embedded in a web of larger collectives—the community, country, planet, universe—and, perhaps, as part of a higher order, however you define it.

As a Mother

Nurturing self and spirit as a mother involves two entirely opposite and seemingly contradictory things: more time to yourself, and more time with your kids. How is this possible? Isn't there a cap on the number of minutes in the day?

In my own life as a mother, I've found that I can pare away excess "stuff" from my daily life to find more time for self-nurturing activities and more quality time with my child. And many of my patients say they've made similar changes. In this realm, too, self-nurture in solitude and in relationship actually feed one another. For when we allow ourselves to recharge and revitalize, the stronger and more centered we are as mothers.

This does not mean that I advise mothers to allot copious blocks of time for what many would consider self-indulgence—expensive shopping sprees, cosmetic makeovers, and so on—at the expense of time spent with their children. Rather, they can achieve a better balance between time spent on fun, joyous, or sheerly relaxing activities and time spent with children. I ask mothers to pay even more careful attention to what's on each side of the scale than to whether the two sides exactly balance out. Am I vegging out in front of TV as my only form of relaxation? Vegging out is fine, but what about taking a mindful walk? What about reading a spiritually nourishing work of fiction or nonfiction? (Though I have nothing against trashy novels as a form of relaxation, either.) What about taking a hot bath while listening to Mozart piano sonatas? What about writing down your dreams in the morning?

As we embrace self-nurture, perhaps the hardest task we face is how to take time away from our children legitimately to meet our own needs, and to do so in a way that doesn't make us feel guilty. One helpful hint is to check in with ourselves about our state of mind and heart: Are we so physically depleted or starved for pleasurable activity that we experience child care as a complete drag, a routine with no redeeming emotional or spiritual overtones? If so, seizing time for self-nurture is the greatest favor we can do not only for ourselves but for our families. Two operative affirmations include, "I deserve to care for myself" and "My family deserves to have me take care of myself."

On the side of the scale representing the time we actually spend with our children, we can also take actions to transform the joyless daily grind.

You know what I mean—shuttling kids to and from school, friends' homes, and extracurricular activities; shopping and preparing meals; cleaning up; ironing out problems with siblings; and other minutiae— the micromanaging of our children's lives inherent in our job descriptions as "mothers." There are two ways to change how we spend and experience time with our children. Rarely can we significantly reduce the amount of time spent on micromanagement, but we can relate to these activities differently. Here, mindfulness can be the most enduringly helpful form of spiritual self-nurture for parents. The country's leading teacher of mindfulness, Jon Kabat-Zinn, has devoted an entire book, *Everyday Blessings*, to mindful parenting, and we can all take a page from his philosophy. He teaches parents how to slow down and pay exquisite attention to the smallest events—from the evening bath to school artwork lessons to cuddling on the sofa. Kabat-Zinn advocates a regular practice of mindfulness meditation, but parents ought to bring that same quality of attentiveness to life with children. Mindfulness practice can enable mothers to experience the mundanities of child care as far less burdensome and more frequently joyous.

One of my patients, Susan, told me she dreaded preparing dinner for her children, which she experienced as the height of drudgery. Making a salad, she said, was pure torture—tedious, time-consuming, utterly without payoff. (How many kids compliment their parents on the beautiful salad?) I suggested that she entirely reframe making a salad by doing it mindfully, with her senses fully engaged in every moment. Susan was skeptical, but later reported a surprising change. For the first time, she saw the vibrant, bright colors of the red peppers, orange carrots, and green lettuce, and heard the crunch and snap of the vegetables as she diced them on her cutting board. By the time she was finished, Susan was delighted by the beauty she'd created: the sensual shape of Romaine lettuce, the mélange of gorgeous greens, reds, yellows, and purples in her salad bowl. In the future, Susan may not always be as entranced by salad making, but by continuing to practice mindfulness, she will never again be as bored and resentful.

The same principle applies to activities with children. If we become more mindful with our kids, we'll recognize just how mindful *they* are— how their responses to everyday events are so often filled with wonder. And we'll be filled with gratitude at their reactions to small events, such as a triumph in the school yard, an off-the-cuff insight into a guest, the joy over mastering a homework problem or difficult game, a show of compassion toward a friend who is hurt. We also nurture self and spirit by letting ourselves off the hook after our inevitable foul-ups and misdeeds. Forgetting an after-school pickup, losing our temper over a poor grade, temporarily favoring one child over another—these typical mistakes are worthy of self-analysis, not self-blame. Unless we are mothers who need to work through a deeper ambivalence about parenthood, a problem that would require counseling or therapy, then we can and should apply this affirmation after every misstep: "I'm doing the best I can."

But we can do more than restructure our experience of the daily flow of events with our children. We can actually create new kinds of experiences by choosing activities with our kids that we and they both love. This requires your willingness as a parent to "get down" with your children, joining them (temporarily) on their level, connecting with the child part of yourself that was tickled by the sheer abandon of a snowball fight, a game of badminton in the backyard, a gentle wrestling match on the floor, or a summer night of hide-and-go-seek. Recently, my two-year-old daughter Sarah and I discovered a song on a Sesame Street video called "Ba Ba Bamba," a great tune with a funky, danceable beat. As soon as I pop in the video, Sarah jumps up and we dance together in a silly way that inevitably leaves us in gales of giddy laughter. When mothers can re-create that childhood state of unadulterated joy with their own children, they've found a common language—the language of play. In such uninhibited moments, the nurturing of self and child come together, and we sense the possibility that everyone's needs can be met.

Spring

A Time for
Renewal

4

THE SACRED BODY:

FROM SHAME TO CELEBRATION

The body's life is the life of sensations and emotions. The body feels real hunger, real thirst, real joy in the sun or snow, real pleasure in the smell of roses or the look of a lilac bush; real anger, real sorrow, real tenderness, real warmth, real passion, real hate, real grief. All the emotions belong to the body and are only recognized by the mind.

—D. H. Lawrence

IN MY WORK with women who are stressed-out, burned-out, infertile, or suffering with illness, I have never met a woman who has convincingly told me that she loves or is comfortable with her body. The majority actively dislike their bodies or have serious complaints about one characteristic or body part; the rest have a vague discontent about their appearance, health, or sexuality. Those of us beset by some form of chronic dissatisfaction should ask ourselves whether alienation from our bodies is the underlying cause. Whether we feel sexually unattractive, overweight, fatigued, troubled by physical symptoms, or obsessed with food, our self-esteem is often decimated by harsh negative feelings about our bodies.

The healing solution is to nurture our bodies. One friend, Priscilla, a thirty-eight-year-old publicist for a media outlet, had struggled with weight since she was a teenager. Like ocean waves, her self-esteem would dramatically rise or fall on the basis of her body image. At odds with her own body, Priscilla experienced sexual insecurities, physical symptoms including back pain and food allergies, and grave difficulties sustaining a gratifying, loving relationship with a man. Here is how Priscilla describes the changes that freed her from the prison of bodily self-doubts:

> A few years ago, I realized just how miserable I felt about my body. I'd been on every diet, gone the fitness route, working out like crazy almost every day. I had moments where I felt okay about my shape, but it never lasted long or went very deep. I realized that my whole self-image would wax and wane depending on my fat situation. This began to make no sense to me. My therapist helped with this. She said, "If fat is going to be your barometer of self-love, you're not tackling the underlying issues. Even if you had your body sculpted, you'd still find ways to feel bad about yourself." So I tried to move away from obsessiveness about fat and tried to embrace my body as it is in any moment. I had to use meditation, imagery, and even prayer to accomplish this. Deep breathing made a huge difference; I realized that I did not breathe into my belly for fear of it sticking out. My energy improved and I gradually stopped beating myself up on a daily basis. If the body is a temple, I realized, I better treat it like one.

Here Priscilla has captured the essence of body-nurture. We can direct our loving energies toward our bodies as surely as we can direct loving energies toward a spouse, romantic partner, or young child. Yet for most of us, this requires a radical transformation in our mind-sets. This chapter will help you to embrace the sacred body: to move from shame to celebration.

Bodily shame is the basis for so much anxiety, anger, depression, and despair. The culprits are not ourselves but our family upbringings, cultural conditionings, and the messages we're fed by the media about what constitutes beauty and worth in our society. By the same token, the fact the we *can* be victimized by social pressures doesn't mean we must be victims. As adults, we can resist these ubiquitous negative messages and free ourselves from shame about our bodies. But it requires effort and a commitment to nurturing our bodies as we would nurture a dear friend who is suffering.

Think about it. Those of us in baby-boomer or Gen-X demographic categories see ourselves as vastly more enlightened than our parents, who were often encumbered by body-negative attitudes and moral precepts. Most of us know better than to shame a young child about the shape of her body, a few pounds of baby fat, an imperfect facial feature, a penchant for snacks, or a natural interest in her sexual organs. Yet by comparison we are thoroughly unenlightened—even cruel—toward ourselves regarding our own adult bodies. We sigh or swear at the sight of our figures in a mirror; revile every "extra" ounce of fat on our thighs or torsos; admonish ourselves over every food indulgence; and are quick to doubt our sexual worthiness.

Priscilla, who eloquently described her own bodily transformation, used deep breathing, meditation, and prayer to move from shame to celebration. Priscilla's story makes clear that body-nurture does not entail hiring a pricey fitness trainer, spending countless hours on the Stairmaster, or embarking on a strict diet of green vegetables and Evian. I have no problem with women who gain pleasure from intensive exercise and low-fat diets, but too many women confuse these otherwise healthy endeavors with body-nurture. Indeed, some of the least body-nurturing women I know are exercise freaks and diet mavens. True body-nurture absolutely includes physical activity and sound nutrition, but not compulsive exercise and onerous dietary restriction. True body-nurture is also much more than exercise and nutrition. It includes the following actions and ideas:

- deep diaphragmatic breathing
- a regular practice of relaxation
- cognitive restructuring of body-punishing thoughts into thoughts of compassion and forgiveness
- delight in the sensual and sexual pleasures of the body
- a sane, balanced, non-shame-based relationship with food
- health-promoting behaviors, such as stopping smoking, alcohol in moderation, and regular visits to the doctor for preventive care
- a profound regard for the sacredness of the body, including all its functions, imperfections, idiosyncrasies, and wonders.

These methods of body-nurture, and other essential techniques of mind-body medicine, clearly benefit women's health. I have published studies showing that body-based relaxation techniques can significantly reduce the symptoms of severe PMS and menopausal hot flashes. In my infertility research, women who joined a comprehensive mind-body group program experienced marked reductions in anxiety, depression, and other forms of emotional distress. As I reported in *Healing Mind, Healthy Woman,* my colleagues and I also discovered that a surprising percentage of 284 women—44 percent—conceived within six months of completing our program. These were women who had averaged three-and-a-half years of unsuccessful efforts to get pregnant. Though we're still trying to ferret out the biological mechanisms that explain this high percentage, I am convinced that nurturing mind and body has a powerful effect on hormones and other physiologic parameters, and can stimulate healing in a range of medical conditions—including infertility.

The body-nurture program that follows involves four key elements: relaxation, cognitive restructuring, emotional exploration, and practical and pleasurable ways to nourish the spirit in the body. Within each of these sections, I will provide approaches that touch not only on body awareness, but on healthy eating and the promotion of sexual and physical well-being. Whether or not you actually begin a body-nurture program in the springtime, commence in the spirit of spring—a time of renewal.

THE BREATH OF KINDNESS: BODY-BASED RELAXATION

Every method for eliciting the relaxation response is a form of self-nurture for the body. You can ground yourself in your body through all nine methods I've described earlier: breath focus, body scan, progressive muscle relaxation, meditation, mindfulness, guided imagery, autogenic training, yoga, and mini-relaxations. Using the techniques that best suit your individual needs and proclivities will remind you that the body is the route not only to pleasure, but to peace of mind. A tense body generates a tense mind as surely as a tense mind generates a tense body. A regular practice of eliciting the relaxation response teaches us to quiet the mind via the body. Mindfulness meditation, for instance, calms the mind by anchoring our awareness in the breath as it moves in and out of the lungs. At times, trying to steady the mind with yet more mental activity is as counterproductive as trying to put out a bonfire with lighter fluid. Body-based relaxation can soothe the mind.

Body-based relaxation also helps us revise our shaming attitudes toward our bodies. Whether we batter ourselves over food or weight, shame ourselves over sexual desires, or experience our bodies solely as sources of pain or illness, relaxation techniques remind us, on visceral and perhaps even cellular levels, that our bodies can be wellsprings of comfort and wonder. Here are the primary relaxation techniques, and several other body-based practices, such as t'ai chi and qi gong, with notes about *how* and *when* they can best be used for body nurture. (Remember to refer back to Chapter 2 for the basic techniques.) I will also teach you how to use physical exercise as a relaxation and body-nurture technique. In several instances, I offer variations on a particular technique that are custom-tailored for body nurture.

Breath Focus and Mini-Relaxations

Most women who feel stuck hating their bodies and feeling fat do not breathe properly. We dread the sensation that our stomachs protrude, even slightly, so we use our abdominal muscles to flatten our bellies. After years of such holding, which is unconsciously reinforced by every billboard, print ad, and TV commercial of a comely model with a washboard stomach, the process becomes automatic, unconscious. We even start holding in our bellies when we're alone. By holding our stomachs tight, we prevent our diaphragms from freely descending as air moves into the lungs. With the diaphragm stuck in place, we can't fill our lower lungs, which are rich in small blood vessels that carry oxygen to our cells. We don't get sufficient oxygen exchange, which jangles our psychobiological alarm bells and sets in motion the fight-or-flight response. We are thus robbed of energy and trapped in a vicious cycle of shallow breathing and chronic anxiety, which further saps our energy, health, and sexual vitality.

No wonder so many women are exhausted! You can break the cycle of impoverished breathing by recognizing its causes and making efforts to breathe deeply. Like Priscilla, the patient who overcame shallow breathing and self-hatred of the body, you can practice breath focus— expanding your stomach as you let oxygen move deeply into the lower portions of your lungs. You can escape the tyranny of shallow breathing by consciously shifting to deep abdominal breathing, with marked improvements in your mental and physical well-being. You may add a mental affirmation to your breathing practice: You might say, "Peace" or "Calm" or "Let it be" during each in-breath, and "Letting go" on each out-breath.

Mini-Relaxations: Mini-relaxations—short-form versions of breath focus that you can practice anytime, anywhere—are regenerative forms of body nurture. Do a "mini" anytime you feel stressed out and recognize that your breathing is shallow. Consider using minis at work, in the midst of difficult interpersonal interactions, in a crowded subway, as a substitute for compulsive eating—whenever your mind receives signals that your body and breathing are constricted. Let your belly move outward as you allow oxygen to enter deeply into your lower lungs. Your energy, and even your sense of control and confidence, will receive a significant boost.

Body Scan and "Soft Belly" Meditation: Focus lovingly on each body part, from head to toe, as you breathe deeply and relax tensions in your scalp, around the eyes, in your jaw, neck, shoulders, chest, arms, belly, pelvis, legs, and feet. To the best of your ability, bring a gentle awareness and nurturing energy to this process.

The body scan nurtures the body, if practiced in a spirit of "merciful awareness," to borrow a phrase from Stephen Levine, author of many superb books on meditation and healing. Levine also offers an exercise, the "soft belly meditation," that helps to heal the split between mind and body. Soft belly can help women overcome the fear and pain that blocks deep breathing and distorts body awareness. While the body scan does include an element of relaxation for the belly, Levine's soft belly meditation expands and focuses awareness on the abdomen. It is especially useful for women who constrict their bellies as they wittingly or unwittingly strain to meet social standards of beauty, or to cut off painful (or even pleasurable) sensations and emotions. Softening the belly releases the pain, and brings the body back into a merciful and loving awareness—beyond self-loathing, beyond judgment of any kind. It helps to restore deep breathing, the free flow of vital energy, emotional awareness, and sexual aliveness. Here is an adapted version of Levine's soft belly meditation. Read it to yourself before you meditate, or tape record your own voice and use the tape for regular practice.

Soft Belly Meditation
Let your attention come into the body.
Let awareness come to the level of sensation in the body.
Feel the physical sensations of being in the body.
Sensations of the buttocks on the chair or on a pillow.
Sensations of the chest moving, the breath.
Sensations in the neck, the weight of the head.
Feel this body you sit in.
Gradually allow your attention to come to the belly.
And begin to soften the belly.
Make room for the breath in the belly.
Breathing in, belly rises.
Breathing out, belly falls.
Soften to receive the breath down into the belly.
Allow the breath to breathe itself in soft belly.
Each breath softening, opening, releasing.
Inhalation, belly rising, filling with softness.
Exhalation, belly falling, releasing any holding.
Expanding and contracting belly.
Soft belly.
The breath breathing itself in the softness.
Letting go in the belly.
Levels and levels of softness.
So much grief in the belly, so much fear and armoring.
Let it all float in soft belly.
Not hardening to the suffering.
Just letting it be in mercy, in soft belly.
Notice how even a single thought can tense the belly . . .
Letting go with each inhalation, softening the belly.
Letting go with each exhalation, making space.
Each exhalation breathing out the pain.
Letting it go.
Soft belly. Merciful belly.
Levels and levels of softening.
Levels and levels of letting go.
Let all that arises pass through the spaciousness of soft belly.
And let your eyes gently open.
Softening with the eyes wide open to the world.

Progressive Muscle Relaxation (PMR):
Out of the Mind, into the Body

Do you often develop headaches, backaches, a stiff neck, stomachaches, dizziness, fatigue, nagging inflammations, and other chronic symptoms? If so, you may be holding stress in various muscle groups, and you may not even be aware of how much psychic tension you are carrying in your body. If this description resonates with you, consider a regular practice of PMR. The process of consciously tightening muscle groups in every bodily region will alert you to areas of constriction, which you can then release with a "letting go" breath. Gina, a middle-aged nurse who had suffered for years with chronic aches and pains, was flabbergasted by the effects of PMR. "My God, I can't believe how tight my shoulders are all the time." She began a daily practice of PMR and found a shiatsu master who worked on her shoulders twice monthly. The positive gains she received inspired Gina to take care of her body for the first time in her life. A little body awareness can go a long way.

Like the body scan, PMR enables you to attend more sensitively and caringly to each part of your body, and to your body as a whole. PMR is particularly useful for women with racing minds. I often have a racing mind; if my brain activity could be translated onto a computer monitor, the screen would be filled with those multiple pull-down menus—lists within lists within lists. (Buddhists call this "monkey mind.") Having a concrete activity to perform during relaxation practice helps me clear the screen of my mind, redirecting my focus to the body. If you suffer from monkey mind, PMR may be the most nurturing prescription for relaxation and body awareness.

Mindfulness: The Wisdom of the Body

In his book about mindfulness, *Wherever You Go, There You Are,* Jon Kabat-Zinn writes, "What we are interested in in meditation is direct contact with experience itself—whether it is of an in-breath, an out-breath, a sensation or feeling, a sound, an impulse, a thought, a perception, or a judgment." All this requires embodiment—living in one's body, in the moment, here and now. When we lose ourselves in thoughts—clinging to them, or repudiating them—the body gets lost, too. By practicing mindfulness meditation, we allow thoughts to enter and exit the door of consciousness, neither grasping nor disowning them. The result is a gradual liberation from the clutches of monkey mind. When we repeatedly return to the anchor of breath, we return to the body—to a sense of groundedness, sensory awareness, and moment-to-moment aliveness.

Mindful Eating: Compulsive eating, spurred by misery rather than hunger, is mindless eating. By the same token, undereating is an emotional reaction against food that invariably involves complex emotional and social issues. Most common among my patients and friends, however, is cruising the kitchen in search of goodies when they're feeling angry, depressed, or bored.

When we eat compulsively, we're like a hungry rat in a maze sniffing for cheese. As we run into the kitchen, we don't stop to contemplate or agonize over the ramifications of a binge session. Primitive impulses take over, and when we find the right nugget, it makes its way into our stomachs with barely a moment to enjoy its taste. Comedian Carol Leifer tells the story of being single and making a beeline for the fridge after yet another dateless evening. No deliberation is involved in Leifer's quick-wristed action: she grabs a can of Redi-Whip, throws her head back, and jets a mounting swirl of whipped cream straight into her mouth.

The crux of the problem for many women is mindless eating. It's difficult, however, to dispense gobs of whipped cream down your throat when you approach eating mindfully. In my experience, mindful eating is one of the best remedies for women with eating disorders. Mindful eating requires us to take several long, slow, deep breaths before eating a meal or grabbing a snack. Then, we eat slowly and deliberately, with full attention to every taste sensation. In this manner, mindful eating restores purpose and pleasure to our gustatory rituals. The problem with restrictive diets is that they rob us of the pleasures of eating, which are not only legitimate but self-nurturing! I strongly believe that women who reject the oppression of rigid diets while embracing the authentic pleasures of mindful eating will find their way to a balanced, shame-free relationship with food. More on that shortly.

Revisit the mindfulness activity on page 38 for a specific exercise in mindful eating. Practice the exercise, then apply what you've learned to your eating habits. The keys to mindful eating are (a) breathe while you eat! . . . with awareness of each inhalation and exhalation; (b) eat slowly, with deliberation; and (c) enjoy and savor every taste sensation with full awareness. Whatever food you are eating, notice its qualities of taste and texture—whether it's salty or mild, sweet or sour, crunchy or soft or creamy. Let the sensory explosions unfold, with as much attentiveness and as little judgment or haste as possible.

The mindful eating exercise can transform your eating patterns and behaviors. During a binge, compulsive eaters neither taste nor fully enjoy their meals. When we binge, we have little awareness of how our food choices affect our biology—an awareness that should not only be intellectual, but visceral and sensory as well. If our sensorium was truly open while eating, we might enjoy fatty foods from time to time, but we'd never stuff down a huge platter of greasy french fries, eat an entire chocolate mousse cake, or gorge on four slices of pizza at one sitting. Mindful eating may be a better solution for many compulsive eaters than diet pills. It's certainly the most self-nurturing remedy, since it says to our bodies, *I respect your needs and limitations, and I'm not going to override them out of boredom, anxiety, grief, or anger.*

Mindful Sex: In today's frenetic world, men and women alike leave their bodies in the dusty trail of career pursuits, overbooked social schedules, and family responsibilities. Few of us carve out enough time to attend to the body with exercise, massage, and body-based relaxation, so at the end of days filled with ideas, plans, worries, and obligations, we often feel disconnected—more heads than bodies. No wonder we're exhausted; not only do we do too much, we think too much, and our bodies cry out when we neglect them.

It should come as no surprise that our sex lives suffer when we leave our bodies behind in that dusty trail.

How can we have sex when we aren't centered in our bodies? Well, we can, but it's clearly not as satisfying or complete. We can change that by reorienting ourselves in our bodies throughout our days. But we can also approach sex mindfully, restoring our capacity to live in our senses, in the moment, fully present and embodied during lovemaking itself.

As Jon Kabat-Zinn says, mindfulness practice is "simple but not easy," and mindful sex is no exception. Proceed with lovemaking with exquisite slowness and intentionality. Let all your senses come into play, attending to every touch, sight, and smell. Remember to breathe. Many women (and men) report that once they attend to their breathing during sex, they realize that in the past they hadn't been breathing deeply or freely while making love. (That old uneasiness about our bellies sticking out may hamper your breathing during sex. I know women who have this problem even though their husbands have been intimate with their every curve and bulge for years.) And how often do you rush lovemaking, because it's late, you're tired, or you're just so used to a particular routine? You can do it differently, simply by choosing to pay attention— breathe into your belly, go *very* slowly, and lose yourself in every sensation, elongating every moment so it is rife with pleasure.

My patients with infertility typically suffer more than most women from sexual difficulties or disinterest. After months or years of scheduled sex, in which lovemaking loses its spontaneity, partners readily lose their passion for each other. In such cases, I prescribe mindful sex. Women tell me that their sex lives have not only improved, but they've become more passionate and exciting than ever.

One couple, Andrew and Karen, had been dealing with the ravages of infertility for three years. After several miscarriages, Karen, who was then forty, had surgery for an ovarian cyst that was so large it required removal of her ovary. While the loss of one ovary should not render a woman infertile, given her age and history Karen was rightly concerned. Their infertility specialist told the couple they could resume their efforts to get pregnant within a few months after her surgery. A year later, after trying every month, including multiple attempts with hormones and intrauterine insemination, they were about to commence with a cycle of in-vitro fertilization. Recognizing how scared and stressed they had become, they decided to attend one of my weekend infertility workshops.

One of Karen's and Andrew's realizations at the workshop was just how much their sex life had suffered over years of scheduled lovemaking. I talked about mindful sex, and that evening they decided to put the day's lesson into practice. Karen later said that the mere concept of mindful sex had completely reoriented the couple. Where before they had little desire, now they let desire unfold. Where before they had rushed, now they took time to give and receive pleasure—to enjoy every caress, every fragrance, every sight of each other. They took time to breathe—a key to mindful *anything*—during the entire experience. It helped, too, that they were at a remote country resort to participate in a workshop devoted to reclaiming their lives. Mindful sex not only reminded Karen and Andrew of the passion they'd once had, it injected new energy and hope into their struggle to have a child. If they could reignite their lovemaking, anything seemed possible.

Two weeks later, Karen and Andrew called off their scheduled cycle of in-vitro fertilization. No, they had not changed their minds about having children. The cycle was no longer necessary, because Karen was pregnant. Not only was she pregnant, but she and Andrew had figured out that they had conceived during that night of mindful sex at our workshop. Today, their daughter, Marion, is a beautiful, bouncy two-year-old.

Given Karen's age, forty-two, her history of multiple miscarriages, and her lost ovary, the couple consider their medically unassisted pregnancy something of a miracle. They can't help but wonder whether mindful sex played a role. Did something about the way they made love help bring about conception? If so, was the healing physical, psychological, biochemical, hormonal, or spiritual? Karen and Andrew have asked the questions, but they don't have answers. Neither do I, except to say that mindful lovemaking has intrinsic value to couples who have lost their capacity for meaningful lovemaking. We do know, however, that mindfulness, broadly speaking, can have a balancing effect on our biochemistry.

Guided Imagery for Body Awareness

My colleague Margaret Ennis taught me a guided imagery technique, which I have shared with my patients, that promotes body awareness as well as physical health and well-being. "Healing Blue Light Imagery" combines guided imagery with body scan relaxation:

Healing Blue Light Imagery
- Take a few deep breaths, becoming aware of each inhalation and exhalation.
- Imagine that you are sitting outside on a mild evening with a bright full moon in the clear black sky.
- Imagine the bluish moonlight coming down from above and surrounding your head.
- Now visualize this healing blue light entering your body. Feel this gentle light inside your head. Experience this light as warm, accepting, and encompassing.

- Very slowly let the blue light move down from the head into the neck, picturing the light as it moves downward and fills the entire area. (This is not a command, it's a suggestion. If the light doesn't go where you want it to, simply take note and move on.)
- Continue to visualize the blue light moving downward, very gradually, from one bodily region to the next, as follows: head, neck, shoulders, chest, each arm, belly, pelvis, each leg, down to the feet and toes.
- As you picture the light slowly sojourning through the body, pay attention to its movements and qualities. Specifically, observe whether there are areas of the body that the light does not seem to permeate. Notice, too, whether in certain areas the light appears to be some color other than blue. Don't try to change, judge, or analyze what you witness; simply take note and move on.
- After you imagine the light in your feet and toes, visualize the light in your entire body. Let your body fill with the blue light, again observing without judgment any areas that seem empty, or of a different color. Let yourself be at peace as the light shines through your whole body-mind.

Healing Blue Light Imagery is a soothing, illuminating variation on the body scan. Mental images can concretize our efforts to release tensions and bring vital energy and gentle awareness to every part of our being. After you finish each session, return in your mind to these questions: Which areas did not fill with light? Which areas were imbued by a different shade of blue, or a different color altogether? Many of my patients with pelvic pain, endometriosis, or infertility find that blue light does not permeate the pelvic region. Several noted that their pelvic areas were illumined by bright red rather than blue light. Use this guided imagery to identify areas of your body that are hot or cold, numb or inflamed, open or constricted. When you practice the imagery again, keep noting what happens in those areas. Don't force blue light where it does not or cannot go; we can't police healing. Remain a compassionate witness to your own process of discovery and healing. In time, an organic transformation will occur, because our psychobiological systems proceed naturally toward a state of homeostasis, or balance, when we remove obstructions. (Forcing matters usually creates more obstructions than it removes.) If we tenderly encourage and observe this healing

energy, whether we consider it merely a metaphor for biological sub-
stances and cells or an entity unto itself, the light of well-being will
eventually find its way to the hurting or deprived areas of your body.

Exercise as Body Nurture

Exercise is a profoundly body-nurturing activity . . . except as practiced
by most of us most of the time.

Just as many of us eat obsessively, some of us exercise obsessively.
That's not to be confused with love of exercise. Women can become
wonderfully addicted to regular jogging (the endorphin rush of the so-
called "runner's high"), the sheer fun of cycling, the rigors of weight-
training, the heart-pumping pleasures of a treadmill, the triumph of
marathoning. These are positive addictions, if I can use such an oxy-
moron. But too many women guilt themselves into overexercising, resulting in fatigue and body injury.

That said, the physical and psychological health benefits of moderate
exercise can't be overstated. It's good for our metabolism, helping us
maintain a healthy and comfortable body weight. It's good for our
hearts, reducing cholesterol and blood pressure. It's good for our immune systems, boosting natural killer cell activity. It's even good for our
brains, easing depression as effectively, in some studies, as powerful an-
tidepressant medications. That's why we desperately need to achieve a
happy medium in which exercise is a natural part of our daily lives, one
motivated by a desire for its joys and health-giving properties, not by
self-hatred or compulsion.

The Brisk, Mindful Walk: Just as you can eat mindlessly, you can exercise mindlessly. By the same token, you can practice mind*ful* exercise.
While I often recommend a slow, mindful walk for relaxation and centering, you may also practice a speeded-up version that is less deliberate
and peaceful, but just as becalming and much more energizing. I call
this simply the "brisk, mindful walk," and the goal here is to push your
body beyond its usual limits. As you take the brisk, mindful walk, ambu-
late rapidly but not frantically, with concentration and purpose. Here
the focus is more on your physical state than on external sights and
sounds. Attend to sensations: your heart beating faster, the quickening
of your breath; the contractions and slight soreness in your muscles. If

you get lost in anxious or distracting thoughts, keep returning to a focus on your breathing. It may also help to restrict your mental focus by repeating to yourself, "left, right," "left, right" in cadence with each stride.

The Relaxation Response During Exercise: You can incorporate the relaxation response into your exercise routine. While this process does not induce the same physiologic changes as relaxation practiced while sitting in a chair, the repetitive rhythms of exercise lend themselves to achieving a centered, quiescent state of mind.

I have never been addicted to running, but I have one clear memory of achieving the runner's high that results from a burst of pain-moderating brain chemicals called endorphins. It occurred during my two-year hiatus between college and graduate school, a time when I lived with three determined medical students and felt a great deal of internal pressure to make decisions about my career. I recall feeling distressed much of the time, mostly because of this looming uncertainty. During this period, I became interested in fitness, partly because I had never been athletic as a child or adolescent and wanted to be, and partly because a man I was dating made a bet with me that I would never run more than a few miles. Of course, I had to win the bet. So I began a routine of swimming and jogging.

I developed a regular ritual of running two miles for 20 minutes, and gradually my fitness improved. During this time—long before I ever knew about the relaxation response—I remember one run in which I focused on my breath as I ran, aware of this rhythm and nothing else until I began to experience a kind of euphoria. I doubled my usual two miles, running up and down steep hills, feeling my body push beyond its limitations. My typical mental preoccupations about graduate school and my future career faded as my physical motions took on a life of their own. Not only was I feeling no pain, I entered a zone of utter tranquility in the midst of the most strenuous activity, a paradox that I found intriguing. It was only years later that I recalled this 40-minute run and realized that I had unwittingly elicited the relaxation response during exercise, which induced a runner's high and a recognition that I could use exercise to manage stress.

Whether the exercise you choose is running, bicycling, aerobics, swimming, rowing, fast walking, or cross-country skiing, the guidelines for relaxation during exercise are simple:

- Become aware of your breathing and allow this awareness to com-
plement the rhythm of your activity.
- Count or mark repetitive rhythms—"left, right" or "one, two" for
walking and running; or the lap number during each stroke as you
swim (one, one, one; two, two, two, etc.). An alternative is to
rhythmically repeat a focus word ("calm," "peace," "om," "*Ham
Sah*, etc.). You may even choose to repeat a short mantra or prayer.
- Maintain the passive attitude of the "witness"—one who watches
the flow of mental activity as if from afar, with calm detachment. If
distracting thoughts enter your head, notice them and gently return to your awareness on breath, the rhythm of your activity, and
your counting or focus word.

Martha, a patient with high blood pressure and related cardiovascular disorders, was advised to pursue moderate exercise. She bought herself a stationary bicycle but could use it only for 5 minutes before
lapsing into exhaustion. I taught her the steps for eliciting the relaxation
response during exercise, suggesting that she focus on the revolutions of
her feet. The first time Martha tried this approach she stayed on the cycle for 45 minutes. Eliciting relaxation during exercise can result in
breakthroughs for many women who otherwise shun physical activity.

Meditation in Motion: Yoga, Qi Gong, and T'ai Chi

The great spiritual traditions of China, India, and Japan include movement arts that could best be called "meditation in motion." These marvelous systems include, most notably, yoga, qi gong, and t'ai chi.
Meditation in movement can balance your vital energy, or "life force,"
without the external application of needles, herbs, or potions of any
kind. You simply use your body in movement to foster inner control and
tranquility. Each system helps to stimulate circulation, deepen respiration, calm the sympathetic nervous system, improve posture and joint
mobility, and strengthen and tone the entire musculoskeletal system.

Yoga: Many women who've joined our programs for menopausal
symptoms, severe PMS, gynecologic cancers, infertility, or the psychophysical toll of daily hassles, report that yoga is among the most effective
stress-relieving methods they've ever practiced. One reason is the hand-

in-glove integration of mind and body movement during yogic practices. Margaret Ennis, a colleague who has taught yoga to my patients, explains its power for women who feel emotionally or physically incomplete: "The relaxation associated with yoga enables women to experience themselves as whole and complete. It has the power to change thought structures, because it takes them to an expanded yet firmly grounded experience of themselves. With this understanding, they can create their lives anew." See page 42 for a brief overview on yoga, but remember that finding the best class and teacher is paramount.

Qi Gong: Pronounced *"chee gung,"* this ancient Chinese system includes gentle exercise and movement, breathing, and meditation. Its purpose is to revitalize and rebalance the flow of *chi*—the Chinese term for "life energy"—throughout the body. Every morning in China, millions of citizens practice qi gong in city parks and plazas. The first program in Bill Moyers's PBS series, *Healing and the Mind,* showed a group of Chinese people in a Beijing plaza being led by qi gong masters; they appeared to be practicing a slow-motion ballet of exquisite grace and simplicity. According to a number of studies, such regular practice can lower blood pressure and reduce metabolic rate, oxygen demand, and pulse. Sound familiar? My mentor, Herbert Benson, M.D., head of the Division of Behavioral Medicine at the Beth Israel Deaconess Medical Center, has also studied qi gong practice and proven that it does, indeed, evoke the physiological relaxation response, which suggests that its health benefits are authentic.

Kenneth S. Cohen, author of *The Way of Qigong,* is an American master of qi gong, and one of the few Westerners to be ordained as a traditional Taoist priest. Cohen views qi gong practice as a gentle yet powerful form of body nurture. I recommend Cohen's books, audiotapes, and videotapes as excellent introductions to qi gong practice, but also suggest that you locate a class with a teacher trained by a qi gong master.

T'ai Chi: The Japanese system of t'ai chi chuan—t'ai chi, for short—is rooted in Taoism, and based on the Chinese philosophic and medical concepts of yin (female) and yang (male), which ought to be in balance if we're to attain optimal health and well-being. T'ai chi consists of smooth circular motions of the body and limbs, with elbows and knees maintained in a slightly bent position. Although just as gentle in its movements as qi gong, the graceful motions of t'ai chi are somewhat more complex, and the sheer number of variations is far greater. (The so-called "long form" of t'ai chi practice is a series of 108 linked movements; the "yang style" short form consists of 37 postures.) But don't be put off by this complexity; a good t'ai chi teacher will guide you gradually from one series of motions to the next, so you can integrate the movements and maintain your focus on breathing and the cultivation of tranquility.

Choose methods of "meditation in motion" when you find sitting meditations too passive, or when regular exercise does not sufficiently generate the groundedness or serenity you seek. Yoga, qi gong, and t'ai chi offer that "never ending river" of calmness, clarity, equilibrium, and awareness.

NURTURE THE BODY'S MIND

Women are veritable factories of negative thoughts about their bodies. Whether these notions involve body image, weight, health, eating, or sexuality, we can be utterly merciless toward ourselves—cruel in ways that would cause us to become outraged if the same thoughts were voiced about us by anyone else.

Here is a "greatest hits" list of common negative thoughts I've heard about our bodies:

I'm fat.
My thighs are huge.
My wrinkles make me look old.
My breasts are too small.
I can't control my eating.
I'm too short.
I'm going to get breast cancer.
My skin looks terrible.
Every day is a bad hair day.
I'll never be attractive.
I'm ugly.
Men don't see me as sexy.
Because of my weight, I'll never enjoy life.

Do any of these sound familiar? Identify your negative thoughts about any aspect of your body and use the four-question restructuring method (see chapter 2, page 47) with as much diligence and care as you can muster in order to challenge and replace them with thoughts that are both more truthful and compassionate.

Food, Weight, and Body Image

Beth, a forty-two-year-old woman with fibromyalgia (a frustrating pain syndrome characterized by achiness in muscles, tendons, and ligaments), has always struggled with food, weight, and body image. For several years, she's been thirty pounds overweight; when I first met her, this was a source of great distress. "I would love to wear tailored suits," said Beth. "But instead I have to wear stretch pants and big sweaters."

Beth was fed up with her limited wardrobe, her nagging self-consciousness about her stomach, and having to avoid even the most fleeting glimpse of herself in a full-body mirror. She could barely bring herself to get a massage for fear of what the masseuse would think when she disrobed. In time, Beth lost her obsessiveness, if not her weight. Cognitive restructuring was the key to her healing process, which involved restructuring these thoughts: "I can't stop eating" and "I'll never lose weight and feel good about my body."

Where had these stress-inducing thoughts come from? The question forced Beth to examine her family. In early adolescence, she was anorexic; by late adolescence, she was bulimic (bingeing and purging); and by early adulthood, she was mainly overeating. Coincident with her eating problems, Beth began developing physical symptoms including her fibromyalgia. Looking back at her relationship with food, Beth realized how her disorder originated. "I refused to eat because of a power struggle with my mother," said Beth. "I had gotten approval by eating, so initially I rebelled by starving myself. Later, when I wanted to please, I ate more, but purged because I was afraid of being overweight. Finally, I began overeating to assuage my own pain."

Her mother had been severely controlling, judgmental, and punitive. But Beth had used psychotherapy to resolve the pain of her relationship with her mother. It was her mother who made her feel worthless, yet for years she'd explain her feelings of worthlessness to herself with the all-too-simple indictment, "I'm fat." Cognitive restructuring helped Beth pull up the roots of her past and present beliefs and behaviors. The process made it easier for her to live by these restructured thoughts: "I can stop overeating, when I choose to," and "I don't have to let being overweight destroy my self-esteem."

Beth's reframing illustrates a critical point about body image. Notice that she did not change "I'll never lose weight and feel good about my body" to "I can lose weight and feel good about my body." *Making our ability to feel good about our bodies contingent on losing weight is the most pervasive, trickiest self-esteem trap I observe among women.* "I'll only feel good when I lose weight" reinforces the family-based or cultural messages that wounded us in the first place. It says, "I can't be worthwhile or lovable or successful if my body does not fit the standard of beauty laid down by my family or culture." Thus, a cognitive restructuring that masquerades as a positive, healthy commitment to fitness and beauty is just one more self-annihilating slogan.

I have nothing against women losing weight, becoming fit, and feeling good about their efforts and results. Indeed, I applaud them. But we encounter serious problems when we link our self-esteem to these efforts, because few of us will ever conform perfectly to social ideals of beauty, no matter how thin we become or how much money we shell out for cosmetic surgeries. We also set ourselves up for trouble, because today's weight loss often gives way to tomorrow's weight gain, and our self-esteem will vacillate along with the fluctuations of our bathroom scales. It is the height of self-nurture to disconnect weight and self-esteem, a simple-but-not-easy prescription that calls upon us to discern deeper sources of self-love. What do we value our loved ones and friends for? Their body weight? Looks? Hair? We usually value them for their positive personality traits, talents, and spiritual qualities. We can apply these same standards to ourselves, transcending our superficial judgments by revering our own intellectual and spiritual strengths rather than focusing relentlessly on our fleshly features.

Use the following sample restructurings of common negative thoughts about our bodies as templates for your own:

NEGATIVE THOUGHT: "I'm disgustingly fat."
RESTRUCTURED THOUGHT: "There is a gap between how I view myself
                          and how my friends and family view me.

They think I'm a few pounds overweight, not disgustingly fat. They can't all be wrong. I realize that I developed this thought in my family; both parents made too much of weight and appearance, and made cutting remarks whenever my siblings or I put on a few pounds. I can view myself differently and question my automatic harsh thoughts about myself. *More to the point, I am not at my "perfect weight," but I feel good about who I am in my work relationships and spiritual life."*

This is only one scenario, of course. But it touches upon the common problem of body dysmorphic disorder (BDD)—the condition in which women's body image is radically distorted, leading to eating disorders, anxiety, and depression. Cognitive therapy, which includes similar forms of restructuring, can be a highly effective treatment for women with BDD.

Some women are genuinely obese, some are thirty pounds overweight, and some are two pounds overweight but think and feel like a person suffering with extreme obesity. But in almost every instance, women with these conditions engage in cognitive distortions that cause immense emotional suffering.

Cognitive work is not about papering over the truth. A woman who is eighty pounds overweight should not deny that she is obese. Such a condition is not only a psychological issue, it can be a serious health issue, leaving women prone to high cholesterol, high blood pressure, cardiovascular disorders, and diabetes, among other conditions. But using the example above, such women can acknowledge their obesity while rejecting the self-flagellation implied by the word "disgusting."

As with the case of Beth and the above restructuring example, identifying the source of your negative thoughts is critical. How did our families handle food and weight? Was either parent overweight? Obsessed with eating or food restrictions? Harshly judgmental about appearance? How did they feel about their own bodies and weight? Conduct these explorations with empathy for yourself as someone caught in a difficult or dysfunctional family system. You can take responsibility for your obsessive eating patterns or negative body image without inflicting more punishment on yourself for your human frailties.

Health Restructuring

Katherine, a patient with severe PMS, had had a tortured relationship with her mother. Her mother had been overbearing and completely conditional in her demonstrations of love. The stress of Katherine's early years, including her parents' divorce and her father's hospitalization for mental illness, was often more than she could bear. To use the psychiatric term, Katherine "somatized" her feelings into bodily symptoms, which did not mean the symptoms were not real. She had suffered from actual colitis, actual dermatitis, and actual PMS. But her conditions were made worse by psychological conflicts and intense emotions, mainly sadness and fury.

Katherine's negative thought, which had persisted for as long as she could remember, was "I'm damaged goods." It took years of therapy, and an ironclad commitment to self-nurture, to enable her to restructure that thought. In her own words, here is Katherine's restructured version: "Now that I have permitted myself to take good care of myself, I realize that I am *not* broken. I am *not* damaged. I am *not* a fucked-up person who doesn't deserve anything good and true in my life." As she learned to care for herself, her symptoms gradually improved.

Other common negative thoughts about health and wellness involve excessive or unrealistic fears, often driven by a combination of media overload and individual psychic vulnerabilities: "I'm going to get breast cancer." "My menopausal symptoms are going to drive me crazy." "PMS will ruin my relationship." "I'll be tired for the rest of my life."

One surefire way to calm our health-related fears is to consult the doctor when a symptom arises. Why should we remain stuck in dread when we can procure a diagnosis that will likely rule out our nightmare scenarios?

That said, persistent fears require not just medical but also cognitive attention. Where do these thoughts come from? Are they based in reality? Few women realize, for example, that the media's frightening statistic—one in eight women will get breast cancer—does not mean you have such a high risk at any time in your life. One in eight refers to lifetime risk, and the majority of women who get breast cancer are diagnosed well in their twilight years. Perhaps your anxieties began when someone you knew—a close friend or relative—contracted the disease or died from it. By all means, practice breast self-examinations and get regular mammograms; these are nurturing forms of self-protection. But also look deeply into the foundations of your fears.

Here is a sample restructuring for health-related anxieties:

NEGATIVE THOUGHT: "I get sick all the time. There must be something really wrong with me."

RESTRUCTURED THOUGHT: "I actually get four or five respiratory infections every year. I assumed that was a lot, but when I closely questioned friends and relatives I realized it was not that unusual. I assumed that I had a weak immune system, but then I realized that my job, teaching in a daycare program, puts me in close contact with kids who sneeze and cough openly when they're sick. Perhaps my image of myself as weak comes from some other source. My mom did tend to overreact whenever I got ill as a child, which made me feel more vulnerable, not less."

The above is based on my experience with a number of women who viewed themselves as essentially unhealthy. Our perceptions can sometimes become reality, so cognitive work can play a central role in our efforts to get well and stay well. I've talked about how you can restructure fears of breast cancer, which are so pervasive. But what if you've been diagnosed with breast cancer? Here is a restructuring that cancer patients find useful:

NEGATIVE THOUGHT: "I've been diagnosed with breast cancer, and it has spread to a couple of lymph nodes in my arm. I am going to have to

endure horrible chemotherapy with
terrible side effects, and I still may not
survive five years."

RESTRUCTURED THOUGHT: "I've been diagnosed with breast cancer,
and it's a very serious situation, and
chemotherapy will probably be very
hard. But I will seek out other women
with a similar diagnosis who've survived
to remind myself that this is not a death
sentence. Indeed, my doctor told me my
chances were very good for complete
recovery, that recent improvements in
breast cancer treatment make this
outcome more likely. Treatment for side
effects is also better, and I am going to
eat well and treat myself with so much
loving care that I believe I can get
through this difficult time. Perhaps I will
even become stronger, and find new
sources of meaning, as a result of this
struggle."

Note that cognitive restructuring for breast cancer is not a turn to
Pollyannaish positivism. I don't think breast cancer patients, or any
other women with serious diseases, are helped by a brand of positive
thinking that borders on denial. We can accept the reality of a frightening diagnosis without pretending it's not happening, or, at the other extreme, becoming so overwhelmed we can't function. In the example
above, we acknowledge fear and difficulty without succumbing to it, and
we prevent ourselves from collapsing by honoring our ability to heal, to
gain support, to receive the benefits of medical treatment, and to take
proactive steps to enhance our recovery on both emotional and physical
levels.

Sexual Restructuring

Negative thoughts about our bodies are certainly not limited to weight
issues; many women are hounded by shaming, critical inner voices

about our sexuality. Women in my practice often associate their sexual difficulties with negative feelings about weight or physical attractiveness: "My fat/thighs/breasts/looks prevent me from having and enjoying sex." In these cases, body-image distortions may be the crux of the problem. But family traumas, fears, or guilts may also be root causes of sexual problems, which run the gamut from insecurity to disinterest to sexual addictions to frigidity and other physical disorders.

Cognitive restructuring can be used to ferret out the causes of the fear, shame, and unmet needs that underlie most sexual difficulties. Women may feel, "I can't get my needs met," "I'll never appeal to the men I want," "My partner doesn't want me enough," or "I feel too bad about myself to let my desires out." These thoughts can be restructured in the same manner as any other automatic negative beliefs.

Recent research showed that upwards of a third of all women have reported past sexual abuse, though most experts believe that such abuse is vastly underreported and is undoubtedly much higher. The sexual attitudes and functionality of women who have been abused is bound to be affected. Women who are frightened of or addicted to sex may not have been abused, but they owe it to themselves to look into their past and find out, to the best of their ability with responsible therapeutic help, whether or not they were. Women who have been abused may dissociate from their bodies and sexuality, or associate sex with violence and abject powerlessness. How can women care for their sexual selves if their sexual selves scare them to death?

Women who recognize that they've been abused should find therapists and/or support groups that empower them to work through the rage and grief associated with their abuse. While this work can be extremely difficult, it can also be liberating. They can finally cast off the albatross of punishing repetitive thoughts about sexuality—the first step toward an authentically gratifying sex life.

Maria, a thirty-two-year-old graphic designer, had been sexually and physically abused as a child. She used food throughout her adolescence to stuff down her anguished emotions, and as she moved into adulthood she wrestled with serious obesity. When I first met Maria, she was 120 pounds overweight, and beset by intense insecurities about every phase of her life, including her sexuality. I worked with Maria and her husband, George, during couples therapy. I regularly noticed George holding Maria's hand, or tenderly touching her shoulder, or playing with her hair. He clearly couldn't keep his hands off her. In my work with Maria, I shared this observation. "Your husband is simply crazy about you," I remarked. In time, Maria was able to absorb this truth, and she used it to restructure punishing thoughts about her sexuality and attractiveness. Her new mantra: "My husband really is attracted to me, whether I understand it or not!"

Most of my patients have not been abused, but they have been subject to distorted family and cultural attitudes about sex. They experience a subtler version of what abuse victims suffer—shyness, shame, feelings of inadequacy, or the "can't get enough" feeling that fuels addiction. Cognitive work helps them uncover the underlying causes of their negative thoughts about sex and replace them with life-affirming, sex-positive thoughts.

NEGATIVE THOUGHT:	"My partner doesn't want me enough."
RESTRUCTURED THOUGHT:	"There is some truth to this statement, but without delving deeper I distort that truth. He has been preoccupied with work, and perhaps that explains his seeming lack of interest. But I am so quickly convinced that he's lost interest that I'm afraid to express my desires. For all I know, he may feel that *I* have lost interest! I need to open up a much more frank dialogue with my partner, and I may discover just how much I have contributed to this problem. He was certainly wild about me when we first met, and that passion lasted a very long time."

The above restructuring is representative of problems—and potential solutions—that arise in many partnerships and marriages ("The passion is gone," "It must be me," "I'm losing my attractiveness," etc.). Go beneath these surface feelings, then take action—communicate more openly and mobilize your imagination to improve your sex life.

Following the example above, take an opportunity to write down negative thoughts about any aspect of your body, including body image, weight, eating patterns, physical health, and sexuality. Restructure these thoughts with as much discernment and loving kindness as you can muster.

Use the reframing process to unearth the sources of your negative thoughts about sexuality, both present and past. With regard to family origins, ask yourself a series of questions: While growing up, were my parents physically affectionate? Was I aware that they had a sexual relationship? Did my parents and siblings talk freely about sex? Was being naked a major taboo? Was there so much nakedness that I felt uncomfortable? Did my mother consider sex something dirty? A wifely duty? An outgrowth of love and an opportunity for pleasure? What attitudes toward sex did I pick up from my father? Our own attitudes, feelings, and behavior patterns regarding sex often have their basis in the family, and we can trace them in search of self-understanding and insight rather than blame and retribution.

NURTURE THE BODY'S HEART

Emotional experience is grounded in the body, and a healthy emotional life—one of high awareness and the capacity to express emotions in appropriate ways—may depend on how we feel about our bodies. If we relate to our bodies as we would relate to a disloyal friend or a reviled enemy, we undermine not only our physicality but our emotionality, since emotions are experienced in regions of the body—gut feelings, yearnings of the heart, passions of the pelvis, anger in the belly. If we distrust and dislike our bodies, how can we enjoy its sensations and trust its messages? How can we honor the feelings it generates? As Stephen Levine has pointed out, when we stub a toe, we automatically send hate into that toe. Can we not send mercy and kindness into a part of our body that is contracted with agony?

When we try to exercise a fierce and tender concern for our bodies, we run into that unforgiving impediment, shame. Countless experts in feminine psychology, from Judith Rodin to Naomi Wolf to Gloria Steinem, have pointed out that shame can destroy women's self-esteem, and shame about our bodies is often the most crippling kind.

One friend, Lainie, thirty-three, suffered for years with large uterine fibroids. They caused pain, bleeding, fears of cancer, and concerns about her child-bearing capacity. It began to dawn on Lainie that distress about her condition was taking over her life. Not only did her condition drain her physical health, but her anxieties drained her emotional life, disrupting her long-term relationship with a man she loved and preventing her from functioning at her best in her work as a stock trader. As she wrestled with the possibility of a hysterectomy, which would end her future hopes of pregnancy, she became even more furious with her body, feeling that it had presented her with a Sophie's Choice—live in pain or give up children. Lainie finally sought professional help from a psychotherapist to deal with the fallout.

What Lainie discovered was that her emotional responses to her fibroids only exacerbated her suffering. She was angry with her uterus for causing so much pain, ashamed of her bleeding, and anxious about the possibility that her body would betray her further by developing an even more serious disease.

Without therapy, she might have blamed everything on her physical condition ("I wouldn't feel this way if it weren't for the damn fibroids!"). But she went deeper with her therapist, exploring why she didn't have more compassion for her body in its suffering, why she always expected her body to betray her. She found the answers in a close examination of her family life.

Lainie's parents displayed more love and respect toward her two brothers than to her, a disparity that continued well into adulthood. She never felt that either parent valued her as a woman, a feeling later confirmed when her mother and father evidenced no pride over her impressive accomplishments as a stock trader. Lainie also noted that her mother seemed angry that she had not yet provided them with grandchildren, as if Lainie's childbearing capacity belonged more to the family than to her alone.

"I was learning that my family never respected my womanhood, so I didn't respect it much, either," says Lainie. "I definitely turned against my body. When I began struggling with these fibroids, it seemed like proof that my body—especially my female organs—were just a source of trouble. I'm not saying that my negative feelings caused the fibroids. But I reacted to them with so much fear and anger that I know I made the situation worse."

Once she confronted her feelings head-on, she was able to plant the seeds for a new cluster of emotional responses. Guided by her therapist,

Lainie practiced an imagery exercise in which she sent mercy and care, in the form of healing white light, directly into her uterus. The explicit goal was not to vanquish her fibroids but to transform her relationship to her reproductive organs. Previously, the only "messages" she got from her pelvis were negative—pain, anxiety, distress. By sending positive emotional energy into the pelvic area, Lainie gradually began to receive different messages back from this region of her body—relaxation, relief, and reassurance.

It began to dawn on Lainie that she possessed the power to reject and replace the body-negative attitudes bequeathed by her family. In therapy, she expressed her anger about the damage they had caused. (She summed it up this way: "I am sick of carrying these feelings! I'm ready to start loving myself as I am.") As she continued to release this anger, she transformed it into a strong conviction to cultivate compassion and pride regarding her body and its organs, not to mention her sexual identity.

In time, Lanie found that through her therapy, imagery, and a dedicated practice of relaxation, she could partially reduce the pain from her fibroids. She was able to accept that she did not have cancer, and she researched and pursued a medical option that enabled her to resolve her symptoms without losing her reproductive organs. Lainie had limited surgery to remove the fibroids, which resolved her symptoms without the hysterectomy that would have rendered her infertile. Lainie also patched up her relationship with her live-in boyfriend, and she was able to revitalize her sex life. "I declared a truce with my uterus," she said.

Lainie discovered what psychotherapist Alexander Lowen pointed out in his book *Pleasure*: "The normal feelings of the body, which are free from value judgments, are modesty and pride. In his modesty and natural pride, a person expresses his identification with his body and his pleasure and joy in its functioning." Modesty and pride may seem like opposites, but Lowen captures the right balance: We can learn to embrace all aspects of our bodies, every delight and fault, feature and function, not with an inflated vanity but with mercy and respect.

Writing explorations can help women to make the kind of transformation that Lainie experienced—a turning point in the life of the body.

I tell my patients with body-based symptoms and shame to practice the following four-part writing exploration:

1. Write out, in no uncertain terms, what you don't like about your body. Specify the body parts or features that you dislike and why. Be as graphic and clear as possible. Express your thoughts and feelings about the aspects of your body you dislike or disdain. Make no effort to be more kindly toward your body than you feel in this moment. Be as truthful as possible, and if that includes harsh terms, don't censor them.

2. Write what you like about your body. Give yourself every opportunity to focus on body characteristics or features you feel good about. Express your thoughts and feelings about body parts that are sources of pride or pleasure. Consider aspects of your body that you may never have realized you regard with esteem.

3. Write about the origins of your feelings about your body. How did you come to dislike certain aspects of your body? What is the basis for your positive thoughts and feelings? Did you gain a sense of shame or respect about your body from your parents? Siblings? Peers? Teachers? What were your family's attitudes toward bodily experience? If you recall an early event in your life that influenced your attitudes toward your body, write about it.

4. Write what you can do to feel better about your body. Focus on feelings (consciously cultivating more compassion and joy), fantasies (letting your imagination guide you toward changes in diet, exercise, and sexual activity that breed health and pleasure), or specific strategies you can undertake (undertaking body-based treatments, fashion choices, preventive and restorative medical treatments, etc.).

I recommend to patients that they write out what they dislike not to reinforce negative attitudes, obviously, but to encourage them to confront their true feelings, as Lainie did when she entered psychotherapy. Women so often harbor a Pandora's box of dark feelings about their physical selves, and the only way not to be enveloped in darkness is to cast a beam of light into the box. At the same time, women find the process of focusing on their positive physical traits—something they virtually never do—to be unexpectedly and mercifully healing.

The final exercise—writing what you can do to feel better about your body—moves you from emotional exploration to action. Use what you discover as the basis for self-nurture of the body, whether that means getting massages, shiatsu treatments, a new sweater, a makeover, taking luxuriant hot baths, getting medical treatment for physical symptoms, or any other action or adornment that honors the spirit in the body.

Emotional Expression and Health: Elizabeth, a seventy-two-year-old grandmother with a sparkling personality, came to see me for a session about her battle with non-Hodgkin's lymphoma. She was actually feeling good about her health; Elizabeth had responded extremely well to chemotherapy. Her cancer was in complete remission and her doctors were optimistic about her recovery. Elizabeth's biggest concern was the effect on her family of her decision not to follow chemotherapy with radiation treatments.

Elizabeth's decision to bypass radiation had not been made lightly. She spoke with her oncologist, who told her that radiation might not be necessary, though it was standard operating procedure. He suggested that she meet with a radiation oncologist, who did recommend radiation treatments. The specialist explained that radiation could slightly reduce the likelihood of recurrent or residual disease, but it was not clear whether she absolutely needed it. Elizabeth also learned about the potential side effects, which included severe fatigue. After gathering this information, Elizabeth made the conscious choice not to undergo radiation. Her gut feeling was that she was cancer-free and would remain so, without radiation and its debilitating side-effects. If she thought radiation would have offered substantial protection against a recurrence, she'd have done it, but none of the medical experts made a compelling case for it.

Elizabeth was at peace with her decision, and so was her supportive husband, Marvin. But her beloved son, Charlie, and daughter, Maxine, were not. "I spoke to Charlie in Wisconsin," she said. "He strongly felt that I should have radiation. I got these terrible feelings in my heart, stomach, and body. When I hung up the phone, I tried to figure out why I was having these frightening feelings. I realized that it was guilt over not doing what he wanted. I was letting him down."

"I've always been the kind to please other people," Elizabeth said. We examined this issue carefully, and she realized that it was supremely self-nurturing for her to stand by her decision. Yes, she would cause her children some anxiety. But our sessions prompted her to speak more openly about her anxieties, admitting to Charlie and Maxine how hard it had been to brook their disapproval. She also took the opportunity to explain more fully the reasoning behind her choice. While they are still anxious about her recovery, Charlie and Maxine have come to accept her decision. Elizabeth has not had to sacrifice her deepest intuitions about her health in order to please them, or anyone else.

"It was empowering for me to stick with my gut feelings," she told me. Today, she remains cancer-free, and is fully enjoying her leisure time with her husband Marvin.

Elizabeth has been an inspiration to me. It was not only her self-nurturing conviction to stand by her decision that I found so impressive. It was the fearless and open-hearted way that she processed her feelings about her body, her health, and her conflict about pleasing others. She fiercely loves her children, and it was difficult for her to deal with their disapproval. But she grew as a result, and her relationships with both her adult children have only deepened.

Elizabeth's story carries several lessons about self-nurturance and health: the importance of making careful medical decisions on your own behalf; honoring your mind and gut when it comes to your own body; communicating openly with your family about health matters, taking their feelings into account but ultimately relying on your own judgment.

She also recruited their emotional support, an important factor in the prevention and recovery from any illness. The data on social support and health is now overwhelming, but emotional expression is key—if you don't use communication skills to procure support from loved ones, you won't get it. A 1995 Canadian study of breast cancer patients offered proof of the healing power of support-seeking. Epidemiologist Elizabeth Maunsell, Ph.D., and her colleagues followed 224 women with breast cancer confined to the breast or nearby lymph nodes. They asked the patients whether they had confided thoughts and emotions to anyone during the 3 months following surgery. The 7-year survival rate for those with no confidantes was 56 percent. By contrast, the survival rate for those with one confidante was 66 percent, while the rate for those with two or more confidants rose to 76 percent.

In other words, turning to others during a medical crisis is not only self-nurturing, it may actually contribute to physical recovery from disease. This principle was also affirmed in psychiatrist David Spiegel's landmark ten-year study of 86 metastatic breast cancer patients, roughly half of whom participated in group psychotherapy that emphasized emotional expression and group support. Compared with a control group, the patients who joined Spiegel's group lived twice as long—an average of 38 months versus 19 months.

The intertwining of emotional experience and health is now the subject of whole new fields of biomedical research. An intriguing body of evidence suggests that expressing emotion in appropriate, balanced ways—to meet our needs and foster strong social ties—can strengthen our hearts, our immune systems, and our overall resistance to disease. As neuroscientist Candace Pert and her colleauges have written, "The [internal] healing system, in all its multilayered complexity, is strengthened and balanced not simply by 'good' emotions, but by the experience, expression, and cognitive resolution of all emotions."

Emotional Awareness and Eating: Uncovering the emotions behind overeating—or any eating disorder—is a sound initial approach to therapy. Try stopping yourself from your compulsive eating, and pay attention to the thoughts and feelings that arise. Here is a dramatic, poignant description of what, at first, can happen:

> The first time I tried deliberately to hesitate before I ate I found that I was scarcely able to drag myself into my study to grab a pen. The urgency I felt, the pressure of the unknown force, made my hands shake. I wanted to move and act and eat and swallow. I wanted cookies and chocolate and gobs of peanut butter. How could I sit down at my desk, how could I hold paper, scribbling frantic words, trying to understand my hunger? "Stillness," "Silence," "Quiet." That was as far as I got. I tossed the paper aside and moved quickly into the kitchen. My hand on the cupboard, I hesitated briefly; but in that split instant I felt the longing and it was not for food. I ate: chocolate, cookies, gobs of peanut butter. Unthinking now, I opened packages, pushing the food toward my mouth. It was larger even than food, a hunger bigger even than appetite. I never before, so far as I knew, had met this longing as a pure desire. I sat down finally, stuffed and sated, and watched this

longing continue to rise. Something about it terrified me. I could not sit there with it for more than a moment or two. My stomach aching, my mouth puckered with the excess of sweetness, I went back to the cupboard and again I ate. . . . Anything to still this longing, to drive it away, to stuff it down and swallow it whole and annihilate it.

This passage is from *The Hungry Self* by Kim Chernin, who finally tapped the rich vein of childhood memory and emotion that fueled her bottomless hunger. Whether emotional factors in eating derive from past or present traumas, anxiety or anger, grief or longing, we can discover them by paying close attention. Chernin's struggle to get answers down on paper is telling. I believe that writing is perhaps the best way to conduct a searching inventory of the causes and potential cures of eating disorders. If you can stop yourself from bingeing and write down the thoughts and feelings that come up, by all means do so. But if you have trouble with this approach, keep a diary of the emotional and situational precursors of bingeing or binge-and-purge behavior.

Guidelines for an eating diary are simple. Be mindful of your eating patterns and what is going on in your life in the minutes, hours, and days prior to losing control. Do you run for the fridge after a fight with your husband? Do you munch on sugary snacks while under intense work pressure? Did you gain thirty pounds after the death of a parent? Look at short- and long-term trends in your eating patterns, and write them down on a daily basis. Record all your observations, feelings, memories, and insights.

On occasion, there are clear situational or habitual triggers for overeating. On days when I work at home, I often skip lunch so I can catch up on a backlog of phone calls. There have been times when I harbored the misguided thought, "Okay, I'll skip lunch. Maybe I'll take off a pound or two." But I soon realized that on days when I skip lunch, by four o'clock I start raiding the kitchen. I ingest far more calories with my late-afternoon raids than with my usual lunches. I have many patients who overeat because they are literally frightened of being hungry. These are patients with mid-afternoon work meetings who eat huge meals at noon because they fear starvation at three o'clock. While it's not a good idea to put off meals, it's just as harmful to overeat out of excessive fear of hunger. Use the eating diary as a sensitive diagnostic tool regarding your eating patterns and as a first step to developing more nurturing outlets for your unmet needs and emotions.

Befriending the Body: Nurture the Self/Spirit

There is an endless variety of pleasurable and playful ways we can nurture the spirit within the body—the "sensual self" that gets lost in the fray of workaday stressors. Let me count the ways:

Body Treatments
Whole body massage
Deep tissue massage
Shiatsu or acupressure treatments
Hot baths with aromatic oils, bath salts, or bubbles
Steaming hot herbal wrap
Long, luxurious sessions in a whirlpool, sauna, or steam room
Movement classes
Reflexology sessions
Polarity or Reiki therapy
Therapeutic touch
Meditation in movement (yoga, t'ai chi, qi gong)
Restorative facials, pedicures, and manicures (a friend calls these "manic cures")

New Looks and Accessories
Sparkly toenail polish
Sheer, silky, lacy underwear
Ankle bracelets
Funky socks
A fabulous scarf or shawl
A sexy camisole
The coolest sunglasses you can find
A new hair color
A new hair style
Novel shades of lipstick, eyeshadow, and blush
That pair of shoes, boots, or sandals you've been eyeing

Pursue these body treatments, new looks, and accessories in the spirit of pleasure and self-care rather than competitiveness. I am constantly drawing distinctions between the strenuous effort to live up to social standards of beauty and the playful love of the embodied self. If you check in with yourself, you'll know the difference. When you go for a body treatment, facial, haircut, or body shop, whom are you trying to please? Yourself or someone near and dear? Yourself or men on the street? Yourself or your family members?

The Spirit of Health: A few months ago, I was in the shower when I felt a lump under my arm. I immediately started to panic. I darted out of the shower to tell my husband, who was as concerned as I was. Dave suggested that I call my doctor immediately and ask if I could get a quick appointment to have the lump evaluated. My reply? "I'll wait till I get to the office." Dave insisted that I call her right away; maybe I could see her before work. I recall speaking through tears as I made the appointment. Fortunately, they were able to fit me in that morning, and within four hours I had had a mammogram, ultrasound, and a diagnosis: a benign enlarged lymph node. Had I not taken my husband's advice, I would have spent at least one whole day, if not several, in a state of severe emotional distress.

My short story can be an example for women concerned about their health. Recently, I was asked by a magazine reporter what self-nurturing strategies I use myself. I assumed she wanted to know about mind-body techniques, including the relaxation response. As soon as I started to speak, the reporter interrupted me: "Wait, I meant Pap smears and stuff like that." I was surprised, since I had never grouped preventive medical tests in the category of self-nurture.

But the reporter's interruption made me think twice. Pap smears and "stuff like that" are indeed self-nurturing. We rarely think of diagnostic tests—or any contacts with doctors or hospitals—as anything other than anxiety-provoking. But there's the rub—we need to reframe our mind-set about preventive medicine from unpleasant (if not dreadful) obligation to self-affirming action. Making regular visits to our physicians for preventive care and early diagnosis is the height of self-care, even of self-love. We prevent undue anxiety, and we may even prevent a disease that would have threatened our lives had we delayed seeking medical care. Here is a partial list of the most important steps we can take to safeguard our health and well-being:

- Perform regular breast self-examinations.
- Receive a mammogram at least every two years after age forty and every year after fifty, unless a family history of breast cancer dictates more frequent screening.
- Schedule an annual gynecologic exam, including a Pap smear.
- Have your cholesterol and blood pressure checked once a year.
- Determine your risks of osteoporosis and take supplemental calcium.
- Carefully consider the risks and benefits of estrogen replacement.
- Speak to your doctor about any other risks, genetic or otherwise, suggested by your medical and family history (i.e., diabetes, colon cancer, etc.) and schedule tests that could result in early diagnosis.

Other ways to nurture the physical health of the body include:

- Maintain a low-fat diet replete with fresh fruits, vegetables, and whole grains.
- Take a daily multivitamin for general health.
- Engage in regular moderate exercises that bring pleasure and release.
- Elicit the relaxation response daily.
- Take advantage of body-based treatments, massages, dance, and movement.
- Procure emotional support from friends, family, and groups.
- Enjoy regular, mindful sex or self-pleasuring (A recent study suggests that men who have regular sex live longer. We can only hope and pray that women are not on the short end of that equation!)
- Practice mindfulness, openness, and explore the imagination.
- Pursue relationships, work, creative, and spiritual activities that give meaning and purpose.
- Use prayer or meditation, relying on any religious verse, mantra, or personal phrase, to reflect your deepest spiritual yearnings or beliefs.

Eating for Comfort and Pleasure: Our guilt-drenched culture, with its emphasis on thinness, restrictive diets, and the ethos of self-denial, is the root cause of eating disorders among women. I'm not the first to suggest that overcoming eating disorders requires women to break the vicious cycle of bingeing, guilt, and more bingeing. One way to accomplish this, as noted by most antidieting experts, is to abandon traditionally restrictive diets and the self-blame they engender.

Eating can be self-nurturing! Indeed, indulging in those much-reviled comfort foods—the guilty pleasures we both crave and loathe—is perfectly legitimate. I get immense pleasure from baking bread for a weekend gathering of friends. The baking itself is a relaxing process, and the first bite of soft, warm bread with a touch of butter is enormously gratifying.

One of my patients, Linda, is helping to care for her mother, who is dying of cancer. One of Linda's greatest fears is that her mother will die before she can finish passing along all the fabulous recipes that reside only in her head. In their Italian American family, food was symbolic of love and caring. When Linda's mother made a vat of spaghetti with meat sauce, the family felt nurtured, and to this day, the sights, aromas, and tastes associated with her mother's spaghetti evoke the warmth of familial closeness.

Is there something wrong with that? Of course not, unless the family was so dysfunctional that food became a substitute rather than an evocation of nurturance. But, of course, many women do fall prey to addictive patterns, overindulging in sugary or fatty foods while underindulging in nutritious foods. One solution I teach is called the 80/20 plan. Put simply, if 80 percent of the food we eat is nutritious—low-to-moderate fat sources of protein, including fish, chicken, and dairy products; fresh fruits, vegetables, beans, and seeds; whole grains and breads—then we can allow ourselves to enjoy 20 percent that fall outside these categories. In this manner, we can allow ourselves the comfort foods—chocolate chip cookies, cakes, ice cream, and chips—with far less guilt and a clear sense that we have not abandoned our physical health or betrayed our bodies.

The Soul of Sex: Nurturing Sensuality

I'm continually amazed by how many of my patients, regardless of their health or psychological status, are uninterested in sex. "I'm just too tired" and "I'm just too stressed," are the common explanations. Many would rather watch TV or read magazines, on most nights, than make love with their partners. Other women offer an explanation that goes to the heart of the problem this book addresses: "To me, sex has become just one more thing I must do to take care of someone else."

Sex as caretaking? Talk about a turn-off! Yet many women forget their bodies and their sensual capabilities when their whole orientation is duty and responsibility: meeting the demands of their jobs, kids, husbands, parents, friends. Under these circumstances, sexuality "goes south," to quote comedian Richard Lewis. Women's orientation toward meeting others' needs, and the energy drain of daily demands, work together to blunt their sexual interest.

My basic prescriptions for self-nurture often help these women regain their interest in sex. The more they tend to their wishes, grant their bodies needed rest, and affirm their own right to pleasure, the more interest and energy they have for sex. But I have several more targeted measures for nurturing your sensual/sexual self with your partner:

- Change your sex schedule. If tiredness is your usual complaint, consider 11:00 P.M. to 12:00 A.M. the danger zone rather than the pleasure zone. You're asking for trouble when you limit your sexual options to the time frame when you're likely to be most exhausted. Plan your weekend schedules ahead of time with sex in mind. (Yes, you'll sacrifice spontaneity, but planned sex is still better than no sex.) Just after waking up may work, since your energy level is usually higher. On weekdays, you might wake up early enough to make love before your morning gets started, unless you have early-rising kids who make this impossible. Carefully consider whether there is a feasible time before your energy window closes—for some women, it's around 9:30 P.M., when sexual excitement is still a fleeting possibility.
- If you have children, plan for evening or weekend sleepovers that give you and your partner the house/apartment to yourselves. Kids

clearly put a damper on many women's sexual interest; the continuous responsibility, time crunch, and fear that they'll enter the bedroom in "mid-act" are antiaphrodisiacs. If you carve out time for being alone, the chances are greater that your and your partner's desires will resurface and blossom.

- Explore and affirm your own creative sexual impulses. Let go of shame, as best as you can, as you explore your body and its unique sensual qualities. The more you learn about your erogenous zones, the easier it will be to guide your partner in ways that maximize your pleasure. Let masturbation become a training ground for positive transformation in your sex life with your partner.
- Attend to your own needs in bed! This advice may be nothing new, but it's still immensely difficult for many women, and they find it easier to implement when I offer my recommendations in the context of self-nurture. Use the skills of assertive communication to ask for what you want in your sexual relationship with a mate. Many of my patients who've given themselves permission to be more assertive in bed have genuinely revitalized their sex lives. Several have told me that taking the risk to communicate sexual desires opens up new vistas in their partnerships. You can move from sex as caretaking to sex as a truly mutual process of pleasuring and release.

I've talked about the role of mindful sex, one of the most powerful ways to nurture our sensual, sexual selves. Here are additional suggestions for nurturing sexuality:

- Let sexual fantasies enter your guided imagery practice. Giving free reign to your own imagination is a powerful way to nurture your sexual self, as one would water a flowering plant. The liberated sexual mind brings the body along for the ride, helping many women with sexual shyness or sexual dysfunctions to open up.
- Write out your most exciting, provocative sexual fantasies. Don't even think about censoring them! Later, go back and see what you wrote. Which fantasies can you realistically enact with your partner, or with future partners?
- Make love in different parts of your house or apartment, using aromatic body lotions or oils, fantasizing out loud in the midst of

lovemaking. Give yourself permission to use any imaginative approach that brings out your wild side, and that of your partner. (But don't let your partner talk you into doing something that makes you uncomfortable.)

• Use mindfulness practice in sexuality to focus on finding pleasure in every moment as opposed to giving ultimate value to the end result of orgasm.

.　.　.

Most women I know have serious trouble with shame. They fight a war with shame every day of their lives, and the battleground is their own bodies. While they feel shame about their behaviors and capabilities, they are perhaps most shame-ridden about their bodies. This is especially tragic given our feminine birthright as women—beings rooted in nature and grounded in our bodies.

It is hard to be self-nurturing when you're ashamed of your body, and it's hard to love your body when you are not inclined to nurture it. The body-nurturing program in this chapter gives you practical ways to break the cycle of shame.

Can we embrace the sacred body? When it comes to bodily experience, can we move from shame to celebration? The spirit of self-nurture offers a way of transformation. As physician Larry Dossey has written, "The power of love to change bodies is legendary, built into folklore, common sense, and everyday experience. Love moves the flesh, it pushes matter around. . . . Throughout history, 'tender, loving care' has uniformly been recognized as a valuable element in healing." We should not only consider the love we receive from others as healing, but also the love we give ourselves, including the kindness with which we treat our bodies.

5

LOVE MATES:

SELF-NURTURE WITH (OR WITHOUT)

SIGNIFICANT OTHERS

✿ ✿

AFTER A DIVORCE and several failed relationships, Marjorie finally found a man who could meet her needs. Gordon was bright, funny, darkly attractive, and caring. The axiom "too good to be true" rang in her mind, but Gordon was sufficiently imperfect to remind her that he was human, not a man who wore a false mask of infallibility. This helped Marjorie to trust him, and trust had not been a big part of her marriage or her other relationships with men.

But there was a problem. Marjorie lived in Boston, and Gordon lived in Winnipeg, Canada, where they met while she was visiting her family. Gordon would soon move to Boston so they could live together before getting married, but in the interim, Marjorie was working overtime to complete her doctoral dissertation in biochemistry at Boston University. Though they found the distance troublesome, the couple maintained their intimacy in long, late-night phone conversations. Still, Gordon was lonely without her, and he begged Marjorie to let him come to Boston more often for weekend visits, and to speed up the date of his move. While Marjorie also missed Gordon, she knew that frequent visits and a precipitous move to Boston would prove difficult for her. His presence would divide her attention when she most needed to submerge herself in her writing. Marjorie was under intense pressure to finish her dissertation, and she'd be unable to find a decent position as an academic researcher without her doctorate in hand.

Marjorie repeatedly told Gordon, "I'm sorry, but the sooner I finish my dissertation, the sooner I can get on with my career and we can get on with our lives. I have to put my needs first in the short-term so that both our needs can be met in the long-term." Marjorie's insistence strained the one intimate relationship of her life that was genuinely nourishing. Gordon felt rebuffed, assuming that if Marjorie shared his passionate love she'd find a way to carve out more time for him. But she made clear to Gordon that she needed to finish her dissertation before she could devote herself completely to their relationship.

Gordon soon came to understand Marjorie's convictions. In time, he was able to say that he missed her without turning that expression into pressure, and she was able to hear his yearning without feeling goaded or guilty. In essence, Gordon realized he could set aside his immediate desires in favor of larger intentions—respect for Marjorie's needs and belief in their long-range dreams for the future. And Marjorie learned that self-nurture, practiced with care and awareness, is also relationship-nurture. The couple's negotiation, which for a short time threatened their union, became the basis for a deeper intimacy.

Self-nurture in intimate relationships has two dimensions, and if they could be worded as a pledge spoken to one's mate, it would sound like this: "I will strive to take care of myself in relation to you, and I will strive to take care of us as a couple."

Women can bestow upon themselves a fierce and tender care without pushing away significant others. In fact, women who creatively take care of themselves develop a stronger closeness in love relationships than those who relentlessly sacrifice themselves for their mates. The rigidly self-sacrificing woman brings only a part of herself to the marriage or partnership, and over time she may be further diminished. The self-nurturing woman brings all her facets and strengths to the relationship, not just her capacity to give. She brings her whole self, and with an unconditionally loving partner, that self only becomes richer and more expansive.

SELF-NURTURE IN SOLITUDE AND IN RELATIONSHIPS

Many of my patients come to me for health problems or difficulties coping with stress. I could teach them relaxation techniques and cognitive restructuring and send them on their merry way, and their short-term troubles usually would abate. But I'm not so sure about their long-term troubles. Because I work with my patients on all aspects of their lives, I often discover that these women have partnerships with serious faultlines. In some cases, the women were aware of relationship troubles but did not connect them with their everyday symptoms. In other cases, the women were not even aware of the problems until we brought them into the open together.

Typically, the troubled relationship was both a cause and an effect of everyday stress and symptoms. The healing therefore had to include repair or resolution of the relationship, whether through individual or couples counseling, a commitment to self-nurture, or both. Other women suffered from lack of a mate, and self-nurture helped them develop either a gratifying relationship or a fulfilling singlehood. In this chapter, I will address both women with partners and those who are single.

For women in partnerships, whether straight or gay, married or not, self-nurture helps repair a wide range of conflicts and imbalances. Perhaps it seems contradictory to talk about self-nurture as a healing measure for relationships. One might think that greater commitment to one's partner, not to one's self, would be the answer. When practiced in a balanced fashion, self-nurture empowers women to be more genuinely giving and committed to their partners, not less. That said, while self-nurture is the best medicine for relationship troubles, it is not an easy quick fix.

When Olivia first came to my office, she was suffering with rheumatoid arthritis (RA), an autoimmune disease in which the immune system attacks tissues in the joints and causes painful and debilitating inflammation. RA has a genetic component, but it can be exacerbated by stress, and Olivia was convinced that job pressures were triggering flare-ups of her disease. I taught her relaxation and coping skills, and we came up with a host of ways she could be more self-nurturing. She described her husband, Spencer, as having been wonderfully supportive throughout her ordeals. But when Spencer joined Olivia for one of our therapy sessions, the man sitting across from me did not jibe with Olivia's rosy portrayal. He took a critical tone with her, albeit a muted one, throughout the session. Spencer took issue with Olivia's newfound commitment to time for herself. While he did not come right out and say it, it was easy to read between the lines, "You're taking time away from being with *me*."

While I was surprised to discover that Spencer was not quite the same man Olivia had described, their problem did not surprise me. As I teach women to self-nurture, I often find that their significant others react to their changes with mixtures of resentment, anxiety, irritability, fear, or even retribution. (Many mates celebrate their partners' transformations, but just as many do not.) Like Spencer, they are unhappy with what they perceive as a loss of time for *them*. But on a deeper level, they may be threatened by their partners' burgeoning self-esteem, since it shifts the power dynamics of the relationship. That is why the development of self-nurture can sometimes be a treacherous undertaking. The solution for these women is not to retreat from self-nurture, but to practice a balanced form—nurturing themselves as individuals and as members of a couple.

In *Intimate Partners*, Maggie Scarf articulates a well-known truism of psychologists who work with couples: In the healthiest relationships, each member is able to maintain a highly developed, separate, individual self *and* a desire and capacity for intimacy with the other. In these fortunate partnerships, both people freely and fully express their "self" needs and their closeness needs, and no intrinsic contradiction is experienced between the two seeming opposites. In such relationships, writes Scarf, "autonomy and intimacy are experienced as integrated aspects of each partner's personhood and of the relationship that the two of them share."

Olivia and Spencer needed to move toward acceptance of each others' autonomy and intimacy needs. In particular, Spencer was perturbed by Olivia's recent assertion of her need for a separate self—time and space to nurture herself at home in meditation and with friends outside the home in all sorts of cultural activities. On one level his distress was understandable: intimacy had always been Olivia's number-one priority. Her own needs had taken a backseat from the very start of their relationship. Rather suddenly, in his view, she was rewriting the rules.

I encouraged Olivia to communicate her newfound desires with compassion and respect, recognizing that Spencer would likely come to accept her self-nurturance once he understood that doing so would actually strengthen rather than diminish their closeness. In time, Spencer adjusted to Olivia's transformation, changing his steps to match her new ones in the "dance of intimacy." Their new dance, as it happened, was more graceful and lighthearted than the old one. Spencer began encouraging her to seize time for herself, nearly shocking her with comments like, "Honey, did you do your relaxation today?" and "Didn't you want to take in a movie with your sister?" Olivia would laugh, realize inwardly how happy she was to hear such words, and take her opportunities for self-nurture.

In the age-old dance of intimacy and autonomy, which is often closer to a boxing match than a ballroom encounter, the introduction of self-nurture, while not without risks, is ultimately the best remedy for the awkwardness, mistrust, and downright hostility that sets in when couples lose their balance. But self-care must be pursued both in solitude and in relationship. The quiet practice of meditation, breathing, or mere contemplation helps women build autonomy by reconnecting them with their emotions, creative impulses, and spiritual yearnings. At the same time, self-nurture in relationship builds intimacy. Spending time in strictly pleasurable or spiritually revitalizing activities with your loved one—a classical music concert, a walk in a botanical garden, an afternoon at a spa, a weekend meditation retreat—breeds closeness. When each partner honors the other's need for both an independent self and an intimate togetherness, their dance will be fluid and sometimes even flawless.

NURTURE THE BODY:
TRANQUILITY, PRESENCE, FORGIVENESS

"Meditation and mindfulness have given me a way to self-soothe that I never knew existed," says Andrea, a thirty-seven-year-old corporate executive. "When things between me and my husband get tough, meditation and mindfulness give me a safe place to go within myself." Andrea and her husband Derek were dealing with a host of problems: his physical recovery from a car accident; stress from the pressure-cooker competitiveness of her job; his grief over painfully divisive tensions within his family; their difficulty conceiving a child; and their ongoing struggle to overcome differences in their styles of communicating emotion.

We all face serious issues and challenges at varying times in the natural history of a relationship. Five years from now, Andrea and Derek's list of problems will change; conceivably, all five major problems will be supplanted by an entirely different set. But what Andrea will have five years from now is a constant set of coping skills—a toolbox, if you will—to handle whatever conflicts and stressors arise in her marriage.

Through mindfulness meditation, Andrea now has that "safe place to go" after a difficult fight with Derek. Over time, she's found that her mindfulness practice is changing the way she and Derek relate. One evening when she returned from work, Andrea wanted to talk about a painful conflict that had erupted with her boss, but Derek was too withdrawn to communicate. Instead of lashing out in fury, she went into the second bedroom of their house and spent 20 minutes meditating. Afterward, she realized that she could soothe herself, that it would have been nice to talk to Derek about her troubles but it wasn't always necessary. Her whole perspective changed, and she turned her attention to his emotional state. When she returned from the bedroom, Andrea asked Derek what was bothering *him,* and she discovered that he was in terrible pain from his injuries. He was happily surprised by her empathic concern, and the couple's evening went from potential disaster to calm togetherness.

Andrea can employ an instantly effective stress-reducer right in the middle of a conflict with her husband—the mini-relaxation. "Minis are now a permanent part of my life," she says. When the going between them gets rough, Andrea also takes mindful walks with Derek. They stroll silently together on a waterfront dock near their home, invariably finding greater peace of mind within—and with each other.

Like Andrea, you can employ relaxation techniques to nurture your body/mind with and without your husband or partner. Here are specific suggestions for relaxation techniques you can use when your relationship, or lack of relationship, is a source of stress or anguish.

Mini-Relaxations During Conflict

One of the most useful techniques for nurturing self in relationship is the mini-relaxation, since you can apply it in the midst of conflict. When you and your mate are becoming embroiled in disagreement or strife, practice deep abdominal breathing, counting up from 1 to 4 on each inhalation and down from 4 to 1 on each exhalation. At the same time, you can combine minis with the "Stop/Breathe/Reflect/Choose" approach discussed on page 70 to interpersonal difficulty: (1) Stop talking and take the proverbial step back; (2) practice minis; (3) briefly reflect on your engagement with your partner, asking yourself how you can practice both self-protectiveness and compassion, assertiveness and forgiveness; and (4) choose your words and actions with care.

Using mini-relaxations and the "Stop/Breathe/Reflect/Choose" technique during difficulties with your partner can bring equanimity and compassion into the moment for both of you. This approach clearly nurtures self (by reducing your own stress levels and enhancing your sense of control) and the relationship (by bringing more awareness and kindness to your interactions).

Meditation as Conflict Prevention

Another technique I have taught my patients is to recognize upcoming circumstances that push your buttons as a couple, practicing minis, or even a 20-minute relaxation exercise with an audiotape, ahead of time. For instance, if you and your mate go over your budget on a weekly basis, and it is usually a tension-filled affair, take time out prior to these meetings to practice whatever relaxation method reduces distress and leaves you feeling most centered. This can prevent potential conflicts from spiraling into full-fledged fights or ongoing sources of estrangement. Be sure to identify situations most likely to push those buttons, such as holiday dinners, the "guys" gatherings at your home (e.g., Super Bowl Sunday, card games, etc.), visits from the in-laws—any event that you know will cause trouble.

If you rely on meditation as a preventive, you may use specific words or phrases during inhalation and exhalation that generate tranquility. One simple approach I teach women for this purpose is to say "calm" on the in-breath and "acceptance" on the out-breath. "Calm"/"acceptance," repeated again and again as you breath during meditation, can alter your entire mind-set with your partner.

In the spirit of self-nurture in relationship, you may also consider meditating together. I recommend that you lie together on your bed, each of you listening to the audiotape of your choice or practicing the relaxation technique that works best for you. I know several couples who swear that joint meditation synchronized their states of mind and brought them closer together.

Meditation with "Safe Place" Imagery

This practice can help you find the "safe place" Andrea spoke of, an inner sanctum to which you can retreat when tension reigns in your relationship, or when loneliness associated with singlehood is the cause of much anguish. Use the basic meditation practice and add this "safe place" imagery offered by Jeanne Achterberg, Ph.D., author of *Imagery and Healing,* and her colleagues:

In your imagination, think of a place that is safe and comfortable . . . a place where you can retreat and care for yourself . . . a place where you can go to replenish your body and spirit . . . a place that is absolutely your own, secure and private. . . . You might choose one of the following examples, and then allow yourself to add personal details and touches that make it uniquely your own.

Form a clear image of a pleasant outdoor scene, using all of your senses. Smell the fragrance of the flowers or the ocean breeze. . . . Feel the texture of the surface under your feet. . . . Hear all the sounds in nature, birds singing, wind blowing. . . . See the colors and shapes as you turn full circle to get a complete view of this special place. . . .

Imagine yourself in a beautiful bamboo forest. . . . You are walking down a path through the tall bamboo plants. . . . Hear the rustling of the leaves, moving gently in the breeze. . . . Imagine leaning up against a cluster of strong but flexible bamboo plants. . . . Feel them swaying in the breeze . . .

In your imagination, find yourself in a very special and private room. . . . You can decorate this room any way you wish. . . . See the colors, and reach out and feel the texture of the surfaces in the room. . . . Let this room be a safe and nurturing hideaway, full of color and music and all the things that you need to feel sheltered and cared for . . .

The purpose of the "safe place" imagery is not to escape the responsibility for communicating and working through conflicts with your mate, but rather to enter a psychic space where you can enhance self-awareness and regain your balance. Returning from your "safe place" imagery, you are bound to approach your partner with greater emotional equanimity.

Forgiveness Meditation

Forgiving your spouse or partner for hurts inflicted is, paradoxically, a profound form of self-nurture. While I never push women into forgiving their mates before they have acknowledged and worked through hurt and anger, when practiced at the right time, forgiveness is an essential step toward healing rifts with our loved ones, and it can be nourished in a highly conscious manner—as a meditation in its own right. Joan Borysenko, Robin Cassarjian, and Stephen Levine, three leading experts in the healing of mind, body, and spirit, are ardent advocates of forgiveness as a healing practice. Levine's forgiveness meditation is especially powerful, and I suggest that you consider this practice when you find yourself unable to let go of anger toward your mate, particularly when that anger seems endless and ongoing. When you recognize that you're stuck in rage, try this forgiveness meditation. At first, you may find yourself going through the motions, but with continuing practice, you'll begin to experience genuine forgiveness.

> Begin by slowly bringing into your mind the image of someone for whom you have some resentment. Gently allow a picture, a feeling, a sense of them, to gather there.
>
> Now invite them into your heart just for this moment. Notice whatever fear or anger may arise to limit or deny that entrance and soften gently all about it. No force; just an experiment in truth which invites this person in.
>
> Silently, in your heart, say to this person, "I forgive you."
>
> Open to a sense of their presence and say, "I forgive you for whatever pain you may have caused me in the past, intentionally or unintentionally, through your words, your thoughts, your actions. However you may have caused me pain in the past, I forgive you." Feel for a moment that spaciousness of the heart which always contains the possibility of forgiveness.
>
> Let go of those walls, those curtains of resentment, so that your heart may be free, so that your life may be lighter.

Mindful Activity

As it was for Andrea, mindfulness meditation can be a boon to relationships by grounding each member in the here and now, where problems and issues are more effectively resolved. But mindful activity is another way to practice mindfulness, and it can be an extraordinary way to nurture ourselves as couples.

Awhile ago, my husband and I discovered the perfect remedy when we find ourselves overwhelmed by our mutual work/home/childrearing responsibilities—a mindful walk. We came to find such peace and fulfillment in these walks, in which we ambled silently and deliberately down the streets in our tree-lined neighborhood, that we now take mindful walks almost every day. We open to the sounds, smells, and sights with full awareness, and thus experience the simple joy of being together in nature, with no words, no pressure to resolve issues—no chance of being ripped out of the present. Consider engaging in a range of activities together while practicing mindfulness. "Shut your mouths and open your senses" is the blunt guideline to mindful activities, such as running, making love, hiking, bicycling, or eating meals together. I certainly do not advocate completely eliminating communication, but I know from personal experience and the stories of my patients that being together silently in the present can open avenues of nonverbal communication, deepening the love between you and your partner.

NURTURE THE MIND: A POLICY OF KINDNESS TO SELF AND OTHER

"I deserve someone better."

"He's such a jerk."

"If he loved me, he wouldn't treat me this way."

"I'm not a good enough wife."

"I don't deserve him."

"I'm not attractive enough to keep him."

"I married the wrong person."

"I'll never find someone who's truly right for me."

How can we neutralize such automatic negative thinking about our partners? First, we must recognize how and why we entertain these thoughts. Notice the polarity here—each thought is of either the "He's no good" or "I'm no good" variety. Women tend to dwell in one position or the other, though many of my patients—and many women I know— lurch uncontrollably from one pole to the other, often within the same day or even the same fight with their partners. "He's no good" thoughts accompany emotional states of frustration, anger, and rage; "I'm no good" thoughts accompany states of guilt, self-blame, and low self-esteem. Women can use careful cognitive restructuring—mind-nurture—to question and replace thoughts at both ends of this spectrum and, when needed, to reduce the agonizing swings from lashing out to self-abuse.

Use the four-question cognitive method to identify, understand, question, and restructure these thoughts, which inflict cruel and unusual punishment on your mate and yourself. Here are some sample restructurings:

NEGATIVE THOUGHT: "I'm a lousy wife."

RESTRUCTURED THOUGHT: "I realize now that I am so overloaded at work that when I finally get home I don't have enough time or energy for my husband. I'm not a lousy wife, just a depleted woman! Instead of blaming myself, I should treat myself with greater kindness, become more assertive about refusing extra assignments, and find more time with my husband so I can feel good about myself as a wife."

NEGATIVE THOUGHT: "I deserve someone better."

RESTRUCTURED THOUGHT: "In my heart, I constantly blame my husband for our problems. He's not perfect, but we have financial stresses and difficulties with our children that are not his fault. When he makes mistakes it's easy for me to fantasize that another man would be different, better. But when I search hard for the truth, I discover that it's all too easy for me to fall back on "I deserve better than this." In fact, both my husband and I deserve better than constant negative thoughts about the other."

NEGATIVE THOUGHT: "I deserve someone better."

RESTRUCTURED THOUGHT: "When I ask myself the questions, 'Is this thought true?' and 'Is it logical?' I find myself answering yes. My husband does not treat me well; whenever conflicts arise, which is daily, he becomes verbally abusive. But I do not always call him on his verbal abuse. I am often silent and withdrawn; once in a while I explode. I do not consistently, firmly tell him that unless he stops his verbal abuse and gets counseling, I will leave him. Instead, I harbor the constant negative thought, 'I don't deserve this.' The thought is true, but I do not hear or utilize this truth. Unless I act on it, this thought is only an escape valve for my unhappiness, a kind of muttering under my breath."

The last two restructurings of "I deserve someone better" show how cognitive work, when used to dig out the truth rather than deliver a falsely positive message to the mind, is both demanding and liberating. In the first instance, the thought was not true and needed to be restructured. In the second instance, the thought contained much truth—the hypothetical woman *is* mistreated by her husband. But she did not use this thought to strengthen and nurture herself; she used it as an escape, "a kind of muttering under my breath." Take a long, hard look at your negative thoughts and how you are utilizing—or not utilizing—any truths to either heal and repair a cherished but wounded relationship or to leave an irreparably dysfunctional relationship.

The Life Pattern of Negative Thoughts

I would add an additional question to cognitive restructuring about our love relationships: "Is there a special pattern to when and why these thoughts arise?"

One patient, Marcy, could not escape the recurring thought that her husband, Cary, was a jerk. In moments of repose, Marcy would say that she loved and respected her husband, a successful architect whom she described as intelligent, witty, and a loving father. But her anger had a corrosive effect, bringing out the worst kind of defensiveness in both herself and Cary. I asked her to keep a daily record of the times she had harshly judgmental thoughts about Cary. She placed the first entry in her "jerk diary" when his parents had come for a weekend dinner. By the end of the evening, she was contemplating divorce. He had committed no major crimes; she simply found his behavior off-putting. There it was, she thought—she couldn't stand Cary whenever his parents were present.

But she continued to make entries later that week, with no parents in sight, and she discovered many behaviors she still judged harshly, such as his whining about plans she'd made for the weekend or incessant complaints about his physical problems. But here again, a deceptively simple pattern emerged. Cary only became childish or cranky after 10:00 P.M. In short, his off-putting behavior occurred when he was exhausted! While his crankiness wasn't her fault, Marcy began to see that she exacerbated the problem with her sharp retorts (i.e., "Will you please keep a lid on it!") Once she realized that Cary became cranky after long hours of hard work and postdinner child care, she was able to forgive him. She then initiated simple strategies like getting them to bed earlier, offering him back rubs, and being careful not to push his buttons after 10:00 P.M. These small gestures helped both partners to unwind and reconnect with each other.

Cognitive therapists often refer to what they do as "cognitive-behavioral therapy," which means that you not only restructure negative thoughts, you change behaviors that typically flow from these disordered ideas. When you recognize triggers, like Marcy's realization about Cary's late-night moodiness, you can change your own thinking *and* your actions, letting go of behaviors designed only to change the other person by force.

Your mate's unpleasantness may be triggered by a variety of circumstances, whether the presence of his family, your family, money troubles, visits by one of his particularly obnoxious friends, whatever. Fine-tune your antennae to such triggering events and you'll put your negative thoughts in perspective, or jettison them altogether. Also, be open-minded in searching for your own contribution to the problem. While rejecting self-blame, ask yourself whether your behaviors aggravate or contribute to your partner's moodiness or withdrawal.

My husband Dave and I recently put this technique to work. With our extensive professional responsibilities, and our young child, our plates have been full for several years. We recognized that we'd become occasionally testy with each other. Once we took a hard look at our patterns, we realized that we were more likely to be irritable before and after social situations, especially when there were many events in a short period of time. We'd simply been too social, and the problematic result was obvious—Dave and I hardly had time alone with each other.

So we started cutting back on social obligations, and when we couldn't, we made certain to carve out opportunities to be alone together. Now we take frequent long walks together, and we sometimes rent videos for our young daughter so she can entertain herself while we catch up with each other. As a result, we've been able to return to our playful selves.

You can practice the same form of mind-nurture regarding negative thoughts about yourself in relation to your mate ("I'm not a good enough wife," "I don't deserve him," "I treat him like dirt.") What are your triggers? Do these self-punishing thoughts arise during particular times, events, or the presence of certain others? Keep a diary to answer these questions, and you may be able to let yourself off the hook, and devise common-sense strategies to modify or avoid these triggering circumstances.

The Relationship Quadrant

Perhaps the most effective cognitive method I have found to help couples identify and heal troublesome rifts is the relationship quadrant. It is a marvelous tool, and in my experience all couples with ongoing conflicts can make use of it.

Basically, the relationship quadrant reveals that each individual in a couple has a particular disruptive tendency that most often causes serious trouble when the other person's disruptive tendency is also in play. This creates a quadrant that couples can evaluate to determine precisely those circumstances and mind states that get them into hot water with one another, and then develop simple strategies to prevent them.

James and Paula, a couple who had separated and wished to rebuild their relationship, used the quadrant to begin the process of healing. Here's how the quadrant worked for them. Paula is a wonderful woman, full of warmth and high spirits, who both works full-time and caretakes her two teenage children. But she is also an inveterate helper who will often drop everything to meet the needs of friends or acquaintances in trouble. With all her responsibilities, and her genuine though insatiable helping impulses, Paula at times becomes quite scattered. Her husband, James, is a lawyer who devotes long hours to his job. His key vulnerability is evident during crises at work, which arise fairly frequently and strain his coping capacities. During these times he is tense and needy. When Paula is focused and James is not experiencing a work crisis, the couple is fine. As long as Paula is still focused when James is in a work crisis, he feels that she pays attention to his needs and they experience little friction. If Paula is scattered and James is not in crisis, he can deal with her being unfocused and they rarely fight. If, however, she is scattered when he is in crisis, he feels abandoned and she feels attacked when he expresses his frustration and anger.

Thus, here is Paula's and James's quadrant:

	Paula focused		Paula focused
1		2	
	James calm/no crisis		James tense/work crisis
	Paula scattered		**Paula scattered**
3		4	
	James calm/no crisis		**James tense/work crisis**

Note: plain text=peace; bold=trouble

In other words, the couple was only in trouble when quadrant four was in play, which was, in fact, roughly one-quarter of the time. When I helped James and Paula to recognize and draw their quadrant, they were flabbergasted. All of a sudden, the confusing, inexplicable, even maddening aspects of the relationship finally made sense, eliciting a simultaneous "Wow!" from the two of them. They had uncovered the specific circumstances under which they tore at each other—when he was in work crisis and she was scattered. The rest of the time, they got along rather well. But they recognized a spillover of bad feeling from "Quadrant 4" times, which eroded the quality of their interactions even during otherwise peaceful (Quadrants 1 to 3) periods. That's why it had become harder and harder for James and Paula to ground themselves in the love, attraction, and mutual admiration that had brought them together fifteen years earlier.

In recent sessions, the hope of reunion that was once shattered has returned. Each has a better understanding of the other: James sees the goodness behind Paula's diversions and Paula has empathy for James's work pressures. Moreover, they now know that when they're in Quadrant 4, one or both must agree to alter their behavior. Either James must put his work crisis in perspective and procure more help back at the office, or Paula must put aside her helping to focus more on her husband. In the event of conflict, one must cede to the other based on a calm conversation about whose circumstances at that time are more pressing.

The quadrant has a built-in kindness: Partners in a couple are not pressured to change aspects of their personalities or deeply ingrained behaviors permanently. They must only negotiate temporary change in one when the other is vulnerable by dint of personality or circumstance.

These negotiations are greatly eased by one of the quadrant's wise lessons: three-quarters of the time we're okay; we only have to watch out for the fourth quadrant. If we can do that, we can resolve our differences with intelligence and compassion for each other.

In my years working with couples, I have seen every conceivable variation on the relationship quadrant. Theresa and John were profoundly distressed after John lost his job as a programmer for a large computer company that slashed thousands of jobs during a period of downsizing. John had worked for the corporation for fifteen years and had been attached to his job, coworkers, and the ego gratification he derived from his work. John was grief-stricken, yet Theresa was also distressed, for John, herself, and for their future financial prospects. But at times John was so emotionally overwhelmed that he couldn't take on the challenge of seeking a new job or new possibilities. Theresa veered between tolerance and intolerance, and John alternated between a sad, anxious state and one of hopeful expectation.

Theresa empathized with John, but she was afraid that he'd be unable to take care of them, so she only became intolerant when fear seized hold of her. The couples' Quadrant 4 troubles took over when Theresa was intolerant and John was sad and anxious. Here is the couples' quadrant:

Theresa tolerant **1** John hopeful	Theresa tolerant **2** John sad/anxious
Theresa intolerant/fearful **3** John hopeful	**Theresa intolerant/fearful** **4** **John sad/anxious**

Note: plain text=peace; bold=trouble

Theresa worked hard to become more tolerant when John was grief-stricken, and John tried to set aside his fear and sadness for as long as Theresa was edgy and impatient.

Write out your own relationship quadrant, focusing on recent events and sources of tension. Use the quadrant to let yourselves off the hook as a couple, realizing your strengths as well as your vulnerable areas in relation to your partner. Ask yourself: When do I get testy, irritable, alienated, depressed, or intolerant with my mate, and what word(s) would I use to sum up this vulnerability (e.g., intolerant/fearful, tense/work crisis, scattered)? Then ask: When do I seem immune to my partner's weaknesses, and how would I sum up the strong suit or positive trait that enables me to be so balanced (e.g., calm, focused, hopeful)? Use the terms to create your quadrant; let this chart be your template and guide:

You strength **1** Your Mate strength	You strength **2** Your Mate vulnerability
You vulnerability **3** Your Mate strength	**You vulnerability** **4** **Your Mate vulnerability**

Note: plain text=peace; bold=trouble

Refer to the quadrant itself to identify the precise situations that lead to strife (Quadrant 4) and then negotiate behavioral shifts to defuse the time bomb in the fourth quadrant. Specifically, you and your partner can make a pact that each of you will do your utmost to call upon your strength when the other seems most mired in his or her weakness.

Restructuring Singlehood

Women who are single can reframe the experience, not to eliminate loneliness but to live fully without a partner, to enjoy their freedom, and to create the conditions for a future relationship, should they desire one.

Prior to meeting the man who is now my husband, I'd been dating a guy I was crazy about. After several months, he broke off the relationship and I was devastated. I vividly recall sitting at my desk at work, crying over this man. A coworker, Anne, noticed my tears and asked why I was so sad. I told her what had happened, commenting, "I was utterly happy when I was with him." Then we had this comically repetitive exchange in which Anne kept saying, "He didn't make you happy," while I kept answering "Yes, he did." Then she elaborated. "He brought out a happiness that was already within you. He did not create those emotions, you did." It took a moment for this concept to sink in. Anne continued, "We have all the imaginable joy, sadness, and contentment within us, these feelings are already there. Some people may bring out these emotions more than other people, but they are part of us, lying in wait." I was thunderstruck, and when I look back on her words I rank them among the most significant ever spoken to me.

Whether you've left someone, been left, or simply have been single for a long time and wish you weren't, reconsider your belief that happiness can only come from a man or woman with whom you are in love. While it would be folly to deny the desire for a mate, and the joys of being in love, it would be just as wrong to believe that pleasure and fulfillment are impossibilities without a mate. In my case, after losing the man in question and taking Anne's wisdom to heart, I recovered rather quickly and found myself taking vacations on my own and getting immense pleasure from my work. Soon thereafter, I met the man I would marry. In the years hence, I have experienced a far deeper and more lasting form of happiness than I did with the man who caused so much pain, reinforcing the teaching that no one other than ourselves holds the key to our store of emotional well-being.

When lost in insecurity and low self-esteem, it is easy to swallow the belief that we'll never meet a suitable mate. The longer we remain single, the more convinced we become that we're unworthy or hopelessly unlucky. When caught in this self-reinforcing trap, the best cognitive restructuring is to say to ourselves, "If I can transform the anguished energy I put into finding Mr. Right into positive energy spent on my own personal development and well-being, I will become so much more fulfilled and self-confident that I will be open to the right man when he crosses my path."

The most articulate expression of this cognitive shift comes from psychotherapist Lawrence LeShan, who made the following statement in an interview several years ago:

> Very often people come to me and say, "How can I meet the right person? I'm very lonely. I don't like the singles scene; singles bars are lousy." The personal ads in *New York* magazine are the funniest things I've ever seen. These people come to me and say, "How can I meet the right person?" And I say the answer is very simple: "Stop trying. Make yourself such an interesting person that you thoroughly enjoy your own company and don't give a damn. And, if they come, that's frosting on the cake. Develop those parts of you that you find really fascinating. Find what you enjoy, and then you will be beating them off with a stick!" About 80 percent of the people I tell this to walk away furious. About 20 percent follow it and start having to beat them off with a stick.

Nurture the Emotions:
Wake Up, Open Up, Stand Up

I have learned from years of experience with stressed and suffering women that by nurturing our emotional selves, we can survive just about anything, including the most tortured scenarios with significant others.

A prime example was Alma, a social worker who endured about as much stress as I can imagine. Alma had married Jules, the man she fell in love with as a teenager, and their marriage was sound for many years. Their families, both from the same city in Israel, had been close, and after the marriage their lives were fully intertwined. The trouble began when Alma, in the couple's fervent efforts to have their first child, began having miscarriages. As I tell my patients dealing with miscarriage, the loss of a baby in utero is surely a death, if not of an independent human being, of all the couple's shared dreams of the child expected to come into the world. The couple experiencing a miscarriage must allow themselves to go through a grief process that is not that dissimilar from the one parents who lose an infant must endure.

Alma continued to have miscarriages, and over time, the layer upon layer of grief took its toll on each partner and on the partnership itself. Alma was more readily able to express her grief than Jules was, but the more she sought his support, the more he sought to distract himself. By the time Alma lost her seventh pregnancy, the pain had become intolerable. Jules began blaming her for the losses, and he started drinking excessively in a vain effort to ease his anguish.

The couple separated, but Alma harbored hopes of reconciliation. After fourteen years of marriage to Jules, she still could not conceive of a life without him. But then came the worst blow—the discovery that Jules was having an affair. As if that were not hard enough, the same day she learned about the affair she found out that the woman was pregnant with Jules's child. He would eventually remarry and his new wife would give birth.

Putting back the pieces of her life would be Alma's great challenge, and she entered psychotherapy to work through the multiple losses she had suffered. The losses continued, however, when a new relationship in which she invested much hope fell apart after one year. The man with whom Alma was involved left the relationship for reasons he could hardly articulate, so she was saddled not only with more sadness but with a bewildering sense that she was either jinxed or being punished by fate.

When Alma came to see me, she was being helped by psychotherapy but clearly needed more coping skills to help her rebuild her life and recover her capacity for joy. My first suggestion, in the realm of nurturing emotions, was that she use writing to vent and explore her deepest feelings. This process was immensely therapeutic and healing for Alma, as she articulates in her own words:

Writing has been extremely helpful. It has helped to write when I feel so much pain, when I am really low. I write the pain out, focusing not only on what I am feeling, but also the facts of what has happened.

I have had to process so many different kinds of grief. When I sit down and write it is usually connected to the relationship with my ex-husband. Obviously, the children I lost are very connected to him; thinking about the relationship brings all of this out. What's odd is that I can sit down to write my doctoral dissertation and there are times when I can't write, when I feel I can't go on. Then I sit down and write about my pain, and it helps me become better able to concentrate. Suddenly, I can do my work again.

I am still struggling with all of this, I'm still struggling. But I am beginning to feel that the pain has subsided a bit and I can now talk calmly about these issues. I feel that I have more inner strength, and interestingly, this process has helped me professionally. I am better able to help people. I can feel their pain more. It has made me conscious of how people struggle when they are really depressed. Sometimes the pain is so great you think you are not going to make it. But I am learning to be patient and accept that it is a process, and that I will make it to the other side.

I can cope with other situations better, as well—at work, in other relationships. I am still very much in doubt and puzzled as to how to have a good relationship. It's been very tough, but I feel as though I have made it to the other side.

That Alma has "made it to the other side" is apparent in her most recent conviction: "I adore children," she said. "I always dreamed that I would have a large family. So I am now in the process of putting in papers to adopt a baby." Alma is ready and willing to be a single mother. "In an ideal world, I would like to adopt first and then meet someone who would accept us both." But because she has learned through hard experience that life offers no guarantees, Alma is moving forward with her life and her healing process.

Although not yet involved with someone, Alma's emotional self-nurture is going to enable her to have a healthy relationship. She is taking care of herself in the best sense of that phrase—working through enormous grief, asking the right questions, allowing herself to be puzzled, not pushing herself to find another partner, accepting the validity and pace of her uniquely personal healing process.

Writing Through Relationship Conflict:

As Alma's experience shows us, problems arise among partners in couples when their styles of handling stress and trauma diverge, when communication breaks down under pressure, when the vicissitudes of life intervene in unexpected and bewildering ways. In such circumstances, we must work through our feelings by ourselves and with our partners. Then we must learn and practice forms of communication that nourish the relationship.

I recommend a two-part writing exercise for nurturing emotions regarding intimate relationships. Here are the guidelines:

1. Consider the most recent conflict or fight with your partner, or the one that is causing you the most distress right now. Without any self-censorship, keeping your pen on the paper for 20 minutes, write out your deepest thoughts and emotions about what happened and what still may be happening between you that is causing strife. Let any feelings of sadness, fear, or anger rise to the surface. As you continue writing, consider these questions: What is causing this conflict? Why are we at odds? Why can't we find common ground?

2. Consider the same conflicts and issues, but now write from a different point of view. Put yourself in your partner's shoes, and write what you believe are his or her deepest thoughts and feelings about the problem between you. Consider where he or she is coming from, and write, without judgment, from his or her side of the disagreement or problem.

The purpose of this exercise is, first and foremost, to plumb the depths of your own experience and then to consider, from a clearer perspective, the deeper reasons for problems with your mate. What don't we get about each other? What is he not hearing? What am I not hearing? What differences in how we communicate keep us from understanding each other? Move beyond the somewhat narrow confines of your own needs to consider the needs, limitations, and suffering of your partner. Accept imperfections, and further, understand the reasons for his inability to meet your needs as you wish them met. Only then can we broach the possibility of forgiveness and the tilling of common ground.

The purpose of the second writing exercise is not to squelch hurt and anger; you've already vented these emotions on paper and can continue this process on a regular basis. The purpose is to validate both your own feelings and your loved one's feelings.

The value of such a process was captured, indirectly, in these words from Tennessee Williams, who wrote them in a letter about his play *A Streetcar Named Desire* to director Elia Kazan:

> Nobody sees anybody truly but all through the flaws of their own egos. That is the way we all see each other in life. Vanity, fear, desire, competition—all such distortions within our own egos—condition our vision of those in relation to us. Add to those distortions in our own egos, the corresponding distortions in the egos of others, and you see how cloudy the glass must become through which we look at each other. That's how it is in all living relationships except when there is that rare case of two people who love intensely enough to burn through all those layers of opacity to see each other's naked hearts.

The writing practice paves the way toward more direct communication with your loved one. A recent patient, Jane, experienced a breakdown in communication with her husband after her pregnancy was terminated because amniocentesis revealed severe defects in the fifteen-week-old fetus. In the weeks after the termination, Ben was supportive and emotionally available. But her pain did not rapidly subside. Months later, on what had been the baby's due date, Jane sat alone at home, grieving and angry because Ben was working late, apparently oblivious to the significance of the day.

I urged Jane to find an outlet for her feelings, so she wrote her husband a letter that said, "I need you to care for me and hold me and protect me. You are the only one who can understand how sad I am." Jane courageously read the letter to Ben, who was stunned and moved. He thought he'd been a supportive husband during the crisis period, and he had. But the letter made him realize that, over time, he had insulated himself, ignoring Jane's ongoing sadness and the significance in her mind of the due date. Now Ben understood what had kept them apart, and he responded with compassion and love. Jane's own writing process, and her sharing of the letter, allowed them finally to "see each other's naked hearts."

Writing for Singles

Women who are single for prolonged periods have often had painful past experiences with relationships—spurned advances, quarrelsome couplings, absurd dating adventures, traumatic rejections, breakups, or divorces. Unless they process these experiences and the feelings they evoke, they are bound to repeat the mistakes of the past. The writing technique helps women to work through these memories and the lingering bad taste they leave about intimate relationships or men in general. This enables them to shed their angers and insecurities and get on with their lives with confidence.

One patient, Grace, was severely depressed when we first met, and described the lack of a mate as the prime cause of her unhappiness. A highly regarded teacher, Grace loved her work but had never been married and began to wonder whether, at age thirty-six, there was something wrong with her. I suggested to Grace that she use writing to "let go" of her sorrows, insecurities, angers, and worries about her future.

"It felt like I unloaded a great weight onto the page," she later reported. "I wrote in my notebook every night, which came to feel like my companion."

The change in Grace was dramatic. What she "unloaded" was her tremendous resentment toward men she felt had treated her badly, and a deep well of loneliness. As a result, she felt less emotionally encumbered—lighter and less beholden to the past.

Nine months after she began writing, Grace met Mark, a theater director, at a party. They fell in love, and a year later they married. Grace is convinced that her writing practice enabled her to become involved with Mark. "I had left my emotional baggage at home," she explains. "When I met Mark, I was no longer carrying that burden with me."

Writing or other forms of emotional self-nurture don't have to be seen as one more way to "improve" yourself in order to meet a mate. They can and should be practiced for their intrinsic psychological and spiritual value. But Grace's example illustrates that good things can happen when you "leave your emotional baggage at home." If you're struggling with insecurities, isolation, or anger associated with being single, use the following two writing practices. Start with the first exercise for the first few days, then move on to the second.

1. Write your deepest thoughts and feelings about being single. What experiences have left you feeling anxious, angry, or depressed about relationships? Did you express those feelings at the time, or did you suppress or ignore them? What would you say to the person(s) involved if you could tell them how you feel now?

2. Explore these questions in writing: Can I imagine being single without feeling like a failure and isolating myself? Can I imagine starting a relationship now? If so, what would I need in place to make it work?

Honing Communication with Your Mate

We all know what "bad fighting" is like. We shout past one another, shooting accusations at bullet speed. Then we throw salt on the wounds with more angry words. When we know in our hearts that the relationship has a fundamental soundness, that it is rooted in love, such communication breakdowns are all the sadder, for they can needlessly erode this foundation. By learning and practicing basic communication skills, we uphold and strengthen our partnerships—it's a way of nurturing relationships.

Harriet Goldhor Lerner has developed clear guidelines for healthy, assertive, nonblaming emotional and intellectual communication. These points apply to virtually any relationship, but are particularly relevant to relations with significant others. I have adapted them from Lerner's *The Dance of Anger*:

- Do speak up when an issue is important to you. We don't have to address personally every injustice or irritation. To simply let something go can be an act of maturity. But it is a mistake to stay silent if the cost is to feel bitter, resentful, or unhappy. We de-self ourselves when we fail to take a stand on issues that matter to us.

- Do take time out to think about the problem and to clarify your position. You don't have to "strike while the iron is hot." Before you speak out, ask yourself these questions: "What is it about the situation that makes me angry?" "What is the real issue here?" "What do I want to accomplish?" "Who is responsible for what?" "What, specifically, do I want to change?" When possible, take time to sort out these questions before speaking out.
- Don't use "below-the-belt" tactics. These include: blaming, interpreting, diagnosing, labeling, analyzing, preaching, moralizing, ordering, warning, interrogating, ridiculing, and lecturing.
- Do speak in "I" language. Learn to say, "I think . . ." "I feel . . ." "I want . . ." instead of "You don't . . ." or "You are . . ." A true "I" statement says something about the self without criticizing or blaming the other person and without holding the other person responsible for our feelings or reactions. Watch out for the disguised "you" statements or pseudo-"I" statements (i.e., "I think you are controlling and self-centered").
- Don't tell another person what he thinks or feels or *should* think or feel. If another person gets angry in reaction to a change you make, don't criticize his feelings or tell him he has no right to be angry. Better to say, "I understand that you're angry, and if I were in your shoes perhaps I'd be angry, too. But I've thought it over and this is my decision."

Karen, a pediatric nurse who'd been married to Harvey for twenty years, relied on these guidelines to shift the dynamics of her marriage. They had one daughter they adored, they shared many interests, and they had a network of supportive family members and good friends. Yet Karen was the kind of woman who gave unreservedly to her friends, loved ones, and especially to Harvey. And Harvey was the kind of man who made all the key decisions about the couple's activities—how they'd spend money, where they'd take vacations, even what restaurant to choose. When this incredibly nice, giving, pliant woman came to me, she was ripe for transformation. After two decades, Karen wanted more say in their lives together.

This was not an easy change for Karen. She had had a very strong, authoritarian father who ruled her childhood household. She had, therefore, slipped comfortably into her role with Harvey, and came to believe that their respective marital roles were as they should be. But she could no longer pretend to be satisfied with so little input into decisions. I knew from the beginning that Karen's transformation would have to be gradual, so I started small. "The next time you go out, why don't *you* suggest the restaurant," I said. Even this minimal assertion was difficult for Karen, and I don't exaggerate when I say that we worked on this issue for weeks before she could make her feelings known to Harvey. When she did, he immediately said, "Fine, no problem."

Over time, Karen asserted her needs in many areas of their lives, including more significant decisions, and she relied on careful "I" statements and other communication skills (see above) to reassure Harvey—and herself—that her newfound desires were not threats to the basic stability of the relationship. Harvey was highly responsive, which prompted Karen to have more insight into her past fears and behavior. She realized that she'd projected images of male power and stubbornness, burned into her unconscious by childhood experiences with her father, onto Harvey. While her husband willingly took the decisive role in the family, he was not her distant, stubborn, and uncommunicative father. In fact, he was flexible and open to change. It was a profound lesson for Karen, and since that first seemingly minor but brave challenge to her husband's authority, both members of the couple feel that the relationship has become more flexible, honest, unpredictable, and exciting.

NURTURE THE SELF/SPIRIT:
SOUL IN SOLITUDE AND RELATIONSHIP

"We not only need to know more about ourselves," writes Thomas Moore in his book *Soul Mates*, "we also need to love more of ourselves in an unsentimental way. We need to be close to the movements of soul that run deep and yet have everything to do with the way we act and feel in life. Such love of the soul . . . is the basis for intimacy among people."

We can be close to the movements of soul that run deep in ourselves while doing the same with mates and the relationship itself. Intimacy, in my experience, grows from these efforts, which don't occur all at once but are threaded into the fabric of our lives in partnership and marriage. Nurturing self/spirit in relationship means accepting the imperfect integration of our efforts to love ourselves and love another at the same time.

Here's how this translates: When our relationship is stressed, either due to the grind of daily life or long-standing differences, we must carve out time for solitude so we can reflect, enjoy purely pleasurable or creative pursuits, engage in spiritually or psychologically revitalizing practice, and regroup. But we must also tend to the relationship with loving concern, which encompasses a readiness to share not just emotions but also soul-satisfying experiences: relaxation, art, sensuality, time in nature, romantic getaways, joint spiritual or religious observance. Fitting these efforts together, along with all our other daily responsibilities, is obviously hard. But fit them together we must, as best we can, without holding ourselves to standards of perfect balance and seamless juxtaposition.

Soul in Solitude

Tending to the soul in solitude is a relationship survival skill. My husband and I are good friends with a couple who has an unusual relationship, one that gives each time for tending the soul in solitude. Both are artists, and the man's studio is a half-hour train ride from their apartment. The studio has a pullout couch and kitchenette, and he stays there two nights a week so he can work late. But this also gives the couple two nights apart, which both say is a boon to their relationship. It allows them time to listen to music each likes but the other can't stand. (She loves jazz and can't bear loud rock; he pumps up the volume on old punk records.) The woman is neat and the man is messy; on their evenings apart she can straighten up without getting in his way, and he can exult in the clutter of his studio. She gets antsy when he talks on the phone too much, so he can have long conversations with whomever, whenever he pleases. She goes to sleep early and he's a late-night person, so she has two nights undisturbed, while he can leave the TV and stereo on until the wee hours without causing major marital disruption.

These variances may make them seem like an unlikely couple, but they share as many similarities as differences, and their arrangement offers each enough space so they can be in those parts of themselves that are sources of irritation when they're together. The two-nights-apart plan has only strengthened their relationship, and vastly improved the quality of the five nights they *do* spend together.

Many of us can't forge such an arrangement, so we must find other ways to assert and satisfy our need for self-nurture in solitude. Find times when your partner is out of the house, or if you have enough space, designate a corner of a room where you can be on your own, one that has your books, CDs, and comfortable furniture where you can meditate, relax, read, listen to music.

Here's a list of ways to self-nurture in solitude when you need to re-mind yourself in thought and action that you are, in fact, an individual separate from your mate. This list also applies to single women who can ease their sense of loneliness through intentional acts of self-nurture. Don't limit your imagination to this list, but use it as a launchpad:

- Turn lounging into an art. Find several spots where you can luxu-riate in the rapture of doing nothing. Outside: a hammock, a meadow, or a nearby park. Inside: an attic lair, ratty yet comfort-able old chair, or couch in a basement rec room.
- When feeling disconnected from or neglected by your mate, or lonely without one, stop waiting for someone else to shower you with affection. Buy yourself a bouquet of flowers or a fabulous flowering plant and put it in your bedroom or home office. Pur-chase the very adornment—necklace, pocket book, belt, or pin—you wished he'd give you as a birthday gift.
- Take yourself to the movie of your choice. Consider a matinee, when skimpy crowds make for a quiet theater and the freedom to put your feet up on the seat in front of you.
- Buy yourself exotic bath salts and take a relaxing, long, hot bubble bath. Shut off the lights and place candles around the edge of the tub.
- Take a walk by yourself in a nearby park or meadow. Make it a mindful walk, in which you soak in the input from all your senses, fully in the moment. You may use the time to remember your dreams or to sort out tangles of emotion. Perhaps you'll conjure new dreams, whether of creative projects, career aspirations, hoped-for change in your relationship or friendships, travel to distant places. Or perhaps you'll use the time to clear your mind of all thoughts. Keep moving, keep dreaming.

- Buy yourself a kite and take it on your walk in the park or meadow. New York psychiatrist Larry Amsel notes that kite-flying can be a wondrous exercise in mindfulness. Watch every dip and sway of your brightly colored kite against the blue sky, feel the tug of twine against your fingers, listen to the distant flapping of its sails against the wind.

Affirm Your Relationship

In private meditation, you can use self-spoken affirmations to transcend and heal disruption or strife in your relationship, or feelings of isolation when you are not in a relationship. Select from the following affirmations or make up your own:

> My needs can be met.
> I deserve to be loved, I deserve to be happy.
> May my heart be open to him.
> May his heart be open to me.
> May I accept his weakness and strength as a partner.
> May I accept my weakness and strength as a partner.
> May we be fulfilled together.

Nurture the Partnership I: Acts of Kindness

We can't read the minds of our mates, and though we often sense their desires through intuition and experience, they must still make their needs known, and we must do the same. How often do we skewer our partner when he gives us a gift—say, a clunky piece of jewelry—that we don't need or even want? The gift analogy is apt: most of us would rather receive an item we crave, something we've fantasized about in our private thoughts that our mates would never consider, than something he likes or guesses that we would like. In realms beyond gift-giving, the same principle holds. When we're exhausted or angered by the daily grind, or downright depressed, only we know what act of kindness or practical support from our mate will be helpful. (Sometimes even we don't consciously know what we need.) He may offer to talk when all we want is a backrub. He may offer a backrub when all we want is to talk. In crunch time, we need a simple way to let our loved one know what we need most.

One of my patients taught me a short-cut method for identifying what we need when we're stressed, depressed, or exhausted. I refer to this approach as "acts of kindness." You and your partner can create a list of twenty acts of kindness you would appreciate from one another in times of physical or emotional distress. When either of you hits the wall, you can refer to your list, determine which act of kindness would be most soothing and comforting, and make your request. I even suggest that you preface your request with the code word "kindness," which signals to your partner that you are sufficiently tired or miserable to need special attention. Then you can say which action you desire. Although the "kindness" code word may seem like a gimmick, it works because it signals more than just "honey, do this for me." It's "honey, do this for me because I am over the edge right now, so please take me seriously."

Here is one example of a woman's "acts of kindness" list:

1. Give me a luxurious massage.
2. Prepare dinner and clean up with no help from me whatsoever.
3. Read aloud to me from an inspirational book on spiritual coping.
4. Pick up a video rental of a romantic movie and watch it with me.
5. Buy me a bouquet of fresh-cut flowers.
6. Buy a box of expensive chocolates and have it at the ready.
7. Pick up a bowl of chicken soup and bring it to me in bed, even though I'm not sick.
8. Insist that I stay prone and restful, and do anything and everything to make certain I stay that way for the rest of the day/evening.
9. Sit and listen to me kvetch without saying one word for twenty minutes.
10. Call back my mother/father/sister/brother and tell them I can't come to the phone right now because I am too exhausted.
11. Pour me a glass of chilled wine and bring it here pronto.
12. Take care of the children without any help whatsoever from me.
13. Let me literally cry on your shoulder.
14. Go out and buy me the pair of shoes I've been staring at in the store window for weeks.
15. Pull me out of my misery by taking me for a walk or drive to my favorite park or nature preserve.

16. Allow us to spend the next hour together in blissful silence.
17. Massage my feet while I watch the film of my choice on TV.
18. Take me to my favorite restaurant and act as if we were on an early romantic date.
19. Plant kisses on the back of my neck.
20. Tell me why you were so attracted to me when we first met.

Have the written or typed list ready. It is not only a vehicle for letting your partner know what you need, it serves as a reminder to yourself of what you need when your energy and spirits have been depleted by the assaults of the real world.

Nurture the Partnership II: Acts of Togetherness

These are active ways to nurture the spirit of a relationship, from the glorious (building a country house) to the mundane (cleaning a closet). Planned and executed with a keen awareness that the sole purpose is mutual enjoyment, such endeavors genuinely nourish the soul of the partnership. Here, by category, are examples of acts of togetherness.

Dates: I'm not suggesting that you engage in some retro attempt to revisit postadolescent mating rituals. But we do need, as adults, to consciously reclaim the romantic and often playful spontaneity of evenings or weekends spent together with no friends, family, children, or intrusive responsibilities of any kind. Consider the following suggestions.

- Go out to dinner at a restaurant you both love. If you want to inject a note of youthful romance and surprise, get dressed in separate rooms so you have no idea what the other will wear until you convene in the living room or car.
- Spend a weekend afternoon with your mate at an art museum, or if you live in a city, go gallery hopping. Explore arts you might never have bothered with before but which intrigue both of you—crafts, sculpture, folk art, photography.
- Buy tickets to the most interesting local or regional theater for an entire season of plays or dance performances, and make those evenings special, with dinner before and drinks or coffee afterwards.
- Pick up a catalog for a growth center that offers courses in

self-development, health, meditation, yoga, and spirituality. Find the weekend or week-long course you and your mate mutually agree would be the most potentially soul-satisfying, relaxing, and fun. Make whatever child-care or scheduling arrangements you must to feel completely unfettered while you're away.

Vacations and Getaways: Plan a vacation or getaway mindful of your need to be together, alone, with no peripheral agendas, family obligations, or other encumbrances. As you devise the vacation, return repeatedly to the mantra, "nurture ourselves." Your purpose must be to nurture yourselves as individuals and as a couple; with this guiding light, your vacation or getaway will most likely be regenerative.

I especially recommend to my burned-out or bummed-out couples that they consider getaways—weekend excursions without the kids to the country or warm-weather clime, often planned or implemented at the spur of the moment. As you plan, make a conscious effort to set aside convention. If you live in a city, the easiest and most exciting idea might be to hole up in a nearby hotel—as relatively luxurious as you can afford—for an entire weekend, telling friends and family that you are away together on business. Many downtown hotels have affordable weekend packages.

Bed-and-breakfast (B&B) inns are good choices for country weekends because the settings are often lovely, tranquil, and far from the madding crowd. The rooms often lack phones and TV, which may be exactly what you and your partner need—to tune out the noisy demands of the people in your lives and the world at large (though at some B&Bs you might have to dodge chatty hosts and guests). Dr. Andrew Weil, author of *Spontaneous Healing*, suggests that stressed-out people take extended vacations from news coverage—refusing to read magazines and newspapers or watch TV news. He believes we protect our health and well-being by giving ourselves periodic breaks from the violent, seamy, trashy, cynical, life-negating stories that make up the bulk of local and national news coverage. B&Bs and country inns are good places to go cold turkey from our addictions to the media, and they tend to be less expensive than hotels.

I recommend that you research B&Bs carefully. There are many national and regional guidebooks available in bookstore travel sections. (I particularly like the "Recommended Country Inns" and "Best Places to

Stay In . . ." series.) Find one that suits all your needs, considering issues such as setting, availability of dining, price, local activities (swimming, antiquing, etc.), and the characteristics of the proprietor. If you are like me, you'll watch out for proprietors who may be intrusive, wishing to befriend guests beyond the pleasant civility of being a good host.

Growth and learning centers in rural areas also make for good affordable getaways. Consider a meditation retreat, where you can not only breathe clean air and eat healthy food, but practice deep relaxation with your partner, renewing your commitment to mindfulness and meaning in your daily lives.

Paired Listening: This is a powerful communication exercise that is also a nurturing act of togetherness. The ground rules are simple. You speak about an issue, feeling, or experience of significance. It may concern your relationship, or another subject or relationship. It should be something personal and pressing, rather than a removed subject like politics or movies. Your partner listens without saying a word, but he focuses completely on what you are saying for 5 minutes. Then you switch sides and listen to your partner as he or she speaks for 5 minutes. The purpose is to accustom yourself to speaking freely without interruption, analysis, or argument, and to listen to your mate without interruption, analysis, or argument.

Paired listening enables each of you to feel heard and understood, an experience that grows as you continue the practice.

I also recommend the following variation—what I call *positive paired listening.* Take turns addressing the following three subjects:

- Something you like about your partner you have never told him/her.
- Something you like about yourself you've never told him/her.
- Something you like about your relationship you've never told him/her.

Each of you should speak for about 2 minutes on each subject before giving the other an opportunity. Practice the same uninterrupted speaking/listening as I described in the first exercise. Then move on to the second and third subjects.

Positive paired listening reminds us that our communications must not always involve traumas, tragedies, grudges, or disagreements. When I first tried this exercise in my groups for couples struggling with infertility, a condition that can demoralize even the strongest couples, the results astonished me. Typically, both partners would come out of the room floating on air. Many had not heard such heartfelt expressions from their spouses since before they were married.

Simple Talk About Dreams: One way to nourish the spirit of your partnership is to share your dreams with your mate. But don't overanalyze. In *Soul Mates,* Thomas Moore touches upon the purpose and poetry of dream-sharing with the person you love:

> One simple way to glimpse the genius [in a marriage] is to tell each other one's dreams. For this purpose it isn't necessary to interpret the dream as a whole, but merely to notice the various situations one's spouse finds herself in night after night. Without any overt analysis at a symbolic or mythic level, we might still come to appreciate the less predictable aspects of our partner's soul life. One way to understand the complexity and puzzle of a dream is to see it as a revelation of the soul that is far wider in scope than ordinary life. Simple talk about dreams might introduce partners to the idiosyncratic imagery and themes of each other's souls. Talk about dreams also moves conversation away from rational interpretations and solutions toward a more poetic style of reflection, an important move since the soul is motivated more by poetics than by reason.

Movies That Heal: You can always go to a movie (when you can find a free weeknight or weekend!), but there's nothing necessarily couple-nurturing about that. It may depend, in fact, on the movie itself. What is couple-nurturing, I have found, is to watch movies with content that is specifically uplifting, romantic, or life-affirming. One of my patients had a round of verbal fights with her husband during the holiday season after financial pressures mixed with family tensions rose to a boiling point. The couple was on the verge of a breakdown of some sort when, in desperation, they decided to see *Sense and Sensibility,* starring Emma Thompson, at their local movie house. The story of unrequited love eventually fulfilled was so poignant, and its ending so stirringly optimistic, that the couple left the theater in an astonishingly better mood. Later that evening, they resolved their differences in a calm chat that lasted fifteen minutes.

I'm convinced that certain movies have that magical quality, and most can be rented at your local video store. They transport us to a realm of romance and possibility, which somehow unties the knots you feel caught in as a couple, or help transcend feelings of isolation if you are single and don't want to be. Even tragedies can sometimes make you more appreciative of your own life.

In his book *Anatomy of an Illness*, the late Norman Cousins wrote about movie comedies that promote the healing process in people struggling with illness. Here is a list of films, most with romantic themes, that can have the uncanny power to nourish relationships, to ease loneliness, and to heal interpersonal rifts that no vacation, friend, or therapist can seem to touch.

Morocco (Marlene Dietrich, Gary Cooper), 1930
It Happened One Night (Clark Gable, Claudette Colbert), 1934
Top Hat (Fred Astaire, Ginger Rogers), 1935
Dodsworth (Walter Huston, Mary Astor), 1936
The Awful Truth (Irene Dunne, Cary Grant), 1937
Holiday (Cary Grant, Katharine Hepburn), 1938
Shop Around the Corner (James Stewart, Margaret Sullavan), 1940
The Philadelphia Story (Cary Grant, Katharine Hepburn), 1940
The Lady Eve (Henry Fonda, Barbara Stanwyck), 1941
Casablanca (Humphrey Bogart, Ingrid Bergman), 1942
Letter from an Unknown Woman (Joan Fontaine, Louis Jourdan), 1948
The African Queen (Humphrey Bogart, Katharine Hepburn), 1951
The Quiet Man (John Wayne, Maureen O'Hara), 1952
Roman Holiday (Audrey Hepburn, Gregory Peck), 1953
Sabrina (Humphrey Bogart, Audrey Hepburn), 1954
Funny Face (Fred Astaire, Audrey Hepburn), 1957
An Affair to Remember (Cary Grant, Deborah Kerr), 1957
Love in the Afternoon (Audrey Hepburn, Gary Cooper), 1957
Black Orchid (Sophia Loren, Anthony Quinn), 1959
The Apartment (Jack Lemmon, Shirley MacLaine), 1960
Breakfast at Tiffany's (Audrey Hepburn, George Peppard), 1961
Doctor Zhivago (Julie Christie, Omar Sharif), 1965

A Man and a Woman (Jean-Louis Trintignant, Anouk Aimee), 1967
Blume in Love (George Segal, Susan Anspach), 1973
Annie Hall (Woody Allen, Diane Keaton), 1977
Manhattan (Woody Allen, Mariel Hemingway), 1979
Out of Africa (Meryl Streep, Robert Redford), 1985
Sweet Dreams (Jessica Lange, Ed Harris), 1985
Moonstruck (Cher, Nicolas Cage), 1987
The Accidental Tourist (Geena Davis, William Hurt), 1988
When Harry Met Sally . . . (Billy Crystal, Meg Ryan), 1989
Men Don't Leave (Jessica Lange, Arliss Howard), 1990
Ghost (Demi Moore, Patrick Swayze), 1990
Sleepless in Seattle (Tom Hanks, Meg Ryan), 1993
While You Were Sleeping (Sandra Bulloch, Bill Pullman), 1995
Sense and Sensibility (Emma Thompson, Hugh Grant), 1995
Shakespeare in Love (Gwyneth Paltrow, Joseph Fiennes), 1998
A Walk on the Moon (Diane Lane, Viggo Mortenson), 1999

Love and Let Love: The Guilt-Free Pleasure Zone

No matter what you do or where you go together, you and your partner can follow one fairly simple rule—avoiding some of the worst marital brambles I've ever seen couples fall into. Whether you are spending a Sunday afternoon in front of the TV, a weekend in the country, or a romantic date at a gourmet restaurant, the rule of thumb is "love and let love." Put simply, enjoy your experience with as much gusto, sensuality, and enthusiasm as comes naturally, but you should not expect your partner necessarily to match your excitement, nor should you cajole or even encourage him to try.

One couple I counsel, Harry and Jean, neglected this advice. On vacation in California, the couple was driving down Highway One along the Pacific coastline, with sensational views of steep bluffs over an endless expanse of shimmering seas. Harry's breath was taken away, and he repeatedly said, "Look at those bluffs. Jean, look!" Jean, sitting in the passenger seat, had seen the bluffs; though she, too, thought they were majestic, now she was reading a map. "Honey, I don't want to look right now," she said. "But Jean, how can you not look? Aren't they spectacular?" Soon, Jean found herself making comments like, "Please don't make me look at those bluffs! I don't want to look at those damn bluffs!"

Harry did not know how to enjoy the experience for himself and leave well enough alone with Jean, who would appreciate the views in her own time and her own way.

"Love and let love" applies to both partners and virtually every shared experience of pleasure: movies, hikes, drives, plays, sports, literature, sexual intimacy. We cannot and should not require our companion to love what we love, or to love what we love in the same fashion. My husband, Dave, is a rabid Boston Red Sox fan, which puts him in the same beleaguered camp as millions of other Bostonians. Long ago, when we first attended a few games together at Fenway Park, Dave clearly hoped I would match his level of excitement and fun, and I simply could not. In time, he recognized that getting me to love the Red Sox the way he loved them wasn't happening. Now, we've found a workable compromise. When he wants me to be with him while he watches a crucial game on TV, I read a book and look up once in a while for a particularly compelling instant replay. He's glad we're together while he has a great time, and I'm glad he's not expecting me to react with a passion I don't share.

We need this kind of lightness of being in order to foster the integration of autonomy and intimacy in our marriages and partnerships. "Love and let love" is therefore a guiding principle, one that dashes illusions of perfect synchrony and harmony in intimate relationships while cultivating the conditions for a closeness based on loving regard for our differences. (Yes, we can have wondrous moments of perfect harmony, but we can crush our own and our partner's autonomy with rigid expectations of nonstop compatibility.)

This loving regard can embrace every facet of our being, and our loved one's being. It should encompass our own and our partner's idiosyncrasies, spiritual beliefs, conspicuous imperfections—our brilliant traits as well as shadow sides. There is no cookbook for mutual love and harmony, but nurturing both self and partnership, simultaneously and indivisibly, with as much lightness and open-heartedness as we can conjure moment to moment, is a worthy effort. "For all of us, of whatever religion or nonreligion, a marriage is a sacrament," writes Thomas Moore. "To care for its soul we need to be priests rather than technicians, and to draw from the wellspring of ordinary piety rather than from theory or formula."

Summer

*Free Time for
the Soul*

6

CHILD'S PLAY:

CREATIVITY AND LEISURE

Art is essentially the affirmation, the blessing, and the deification of existence.

—Friedrich Nietzsche

Peace of mind is not a rare and exotic flower that only blooms on deserted islands or on top of mountains. You don't have to travel far and wide to find it. Relaxation is actually a native plant that grows in your own backyard—a hardy one at that.

—Veronique Vienne

WHEN OUR DAYS are filled to overflowing with work pressures, family obligations, and household chores, we start to feel as though we need every ounce of energy and every minute of the day just to get by. At the end of such days, we plop down in our beds as if weighed down by sandbags, and all we can do is stare at the television set, or stare wordlessly at our mates, too tired even to speak. For some of us, such days are so commonplace it's depressing.

When our lives are characterized by this sort of frenzy, we give up a lot. We surrender large tracts of that most precious of contemporary commodities—quality time—with our partners, friends, and children. We often bemoan this loss, but we hardly even recognize that we also sacrifice quality time for ourselves. One of the first and most invaluable possessions we lose when overstressed is time for creativity and leisure.

We impulsively push creative and relaxing pursuits to the bottom of our to-do lists, based on the knee-jerk assumption that they are *always* less important. But it's not enough for me to recommend a reshuffling of priorities; we need to understand why we short-shrift ourselves before we can change. While every woman's history may provide specific reasons, I think that the following generalization holds true: Women have been trained, by families and culture, to feel guilty about taking time for creativity and leisure. We've been taught to fulfill our roles as wives, mothers, and successful career women, and if there's any time left over, we'd better find something "productive" to do. "Productive" doesn't mean painting or singing or taking photographs, and it certainly doesn't mean kicking back with a trashy novel. It means keeping the house squeaky clean, clearing out those cluttered closets, paying those bills, or finding new ways to be certain our loved ones' needs are tended. This training anchors in our unconscious minds, where it dictates our daily choices; hence, pure creativity and "play" often come last in our written and unwritten lists of priorities.

Awhile ago, I was giving a talk on a weekday afternoon that I thought was scheduled to conclude at four o'clock—perfect timing since I was to pick up my three-year-old daughter from day care at five. As it turned out, the talk ended at three, so I had an extra hour. I was left with a choice: pick up my daughter early and spend the hour with her, or head home and spend the hour relaxing. I agonized. My brain paddled the ping-pong back and forth: I'll get Sarah, I'll go home, I'll get Sarah, I'll go home, ad infinitum. Then I remembered that I was writing a book on self-nurture, which finally propelled the thought "I'll go home" to victory. I spent the hour on my porch, reading the paper and listening to the birds chirping. It was a blissful respite, and I picked up Sarah from day care in a much more relaxed state than I had been after my talk. I was acutely aware that I felt more present with her from the moment I saw her at the day care center, and we spent a fun late afternoon and dinner together.

As it happened, a few days later I was scheduled to give a talk at a conference on stress and parenting. I thought the story was a good illustration of how self-nurturance—in this instance, grasping some unadulterated (and unexpected) leisure time—is not only good for ourselves but for our loved ones as well. So I included the anecdote in my remarks to this group of seventy people, the vast majority of whom were mothers. To my astonishment, there were a number of audible gasps when I spoke of my decision to go home rather than pick up my daughter early. One woman bluntly asked, "How could you have done that?" Other women nodded or made sympathetic noises. I defended my choice by emphasizing how much more relaxed, energetic, and present I had been with Sarah, given the hour spent recharging my batteries. I was certain that taking the time made me a better mother that day.

Certainly, the example of choosing to take time for one's self over time with one's child can push buttons for a lot of women. But while women feel most conflicted about pure leisure time—"doing nothing"— some of us feel as bad about time for creative expression. One would think that we'd view creativity as "more productive" and hence less guilt-producing than leisure, yet we still seem to believe that self-expression is less of a priority than satisfying the needs of others. Not only that, but the closer our creativity moves toward play and away from work, the less we may view it as productive and, hence, the less entitled we feel. Our creative instincts are engaged whether we're redecorating our living room or dancing to rock music, but we're not as likely to feel we're wasting time with the former activity as the latter.

Guilt about creative expression is far from the only obstacle we face. Many women—and men, too—make unmerciful judgments or, even worse, prejudgments, about their creative worth. We don't take the first steps toward fulfilling our creativity when we decide we don't have the talent even to begin. Some women believe that pursuing creative expression will not only alienate friends and family, but also make us appear foolish to the world. And we certainly fear failure, but we may also fear success and its consequences.

One friend, Rachel, had always wanted to be a singer of classical music, including opera. After years of fantasizing, she finally got up the nerve to take singing lessons with a top-flight teacher. But Rachel quickly hit a snag. She had a lovely voice, but she had trouble projecting it and her teacher encouraged her to breathe more deeply and open her throat. The more she tried to follow his advice, the thinner and more strained her voice sounded. Her frustration led her to a body-based psychotherapist who taught Rachel to open her throat and let sounds flow out freely, without any demand to produce rich or highly modulated tones. When she did, she began to warble and croon and scream and cry. Afterward, when she talked about the emotions that surfaced with the sounds, she discovered how deeply her fears of failure cut, how much her difficult relationship with her stern father had silenced her, how scared she was of raising her voice. Rachel had always wanted her mellifluous voice to be heard, but her fear had been even stronger. Now, finally, she was able to let her desire to freely sing outweigh her anxiety. Her singing teacher was astonished by her progress; suddenly, her voice rang out with new strength, beauty, and clarity. Rachel went on to establish a successful part-time career singing classical music and arias at concerts around the country.

If we're fortunate, creativity is an intrinsic part of our work lives. All too often, however, work is a far from sufficient vehicle; our deepest creative impulses are too varied and unruly to be given free rein in our jobs. One way to nurture creativity is to develop new means of creative expression on the job; but the other way, honoring the fact that our creativity is larger than our occupation, is to enhance creative expression in our personal lives.

In Lawrence LeShan's words, we can find our own style of being, relating, and creating that makes us glad to get up in the morning, one that feeds our zest and enthusiasm for life. The call to creativity may make us want to sing ballads, paint with gobs of color, slow dance, draw hieroglyphs, make home movies, write short stories, make pottery, or design a country house. Nurturing our creative selves means opening our minds and hearts to the sea of possibilities, to heed the inner voice of imagination.

Play is at the heart of both creative expression and creative leisure. We do ourselves a favor when we recover the spirit of play, not just while on vacation but in our everyday activities, in solitude and relationship, in productive work or totally unproductive recreation.

NURTURE THE BODY: RELAXATION AND PLAY

I'm not too fond of sports analogies, but there's an apt one relating to creativity and leisure. In almost any sport—certainly baseball, basketball, and football—commentators are likely to explain a team's loss by noting that the players seemed "tight." Athletes who can't "get loose" are by definition "uptight," "tense," and "wound up," which leads them to perform awkwardly, without their natural grace or instinctual intelligence.

While professional athletes surely must develop highly evolved skills and a full intellectual grasp of the rules and strategies of a complex game, they must still be able *to play*, to draw on that reservoir of boundless energy and desire for fun that started with childhood games. When we watch premier athletes, we know that their unfettered enthusiasm is no different from when they were kids. (Did you ever see Michael Jordan stick out his tongue as he drove for a layup? He did it almost every time.)

My point here is that every kind of creativity depends on our ability to play. And, in order to play we, too, must be loose. As with sports, the more physical forms of creative expression, such as dancing and singing, require us to be physically loose. But virtually every other mode of artistic expression, whether painting, drawing, writing, filmmaking, or sculpting, calls on us to be mentally loose as well—open to the free play of thoughts, images, feelings, and impulses that bubble up from the unconscious or conscious mind. Indeed, when we have difficulties with creativity, we may be said to be "tight," just like athletes. "Writer's block" is a prime example; every writer who has suffered from this form of creative constipation knows that she is too tense to allow herself to "play" with ideas, words, and images. The critical mind takes over, and the creative mind gets stuck in a prison of doubt and confusion.

Thus, eliciting the relaxation response is a profoundly useful and sometimes even necessary way to revive our capacity for play. Most forms of relaxation help to clear our minds of the cognitive clutter, intrusive thoughts, and critical clap-trap that prevent us from allowing our creative impulses to flow. The more physical techniques—body scan and progressive muscle relaxation—can melt muscular tensions that prevent us from the free bodily expression required to dance, play sports, sing, and practice any form of movement with enjoyment and grace.

Herbert Benson, M.D., has talked about the role of relaxation in learning. "When you are anxious, you can't learn," he has said. "It's like dropping seeds on concrete." The same can be said for creativity. By dissolving mental and muscular tensions, relaxation softens the ground that is the creative mind, allowing images and ideas to blossom.

I know a fiction writer who suffered from such severe writer's block that it threatened her livelihood. Zoe labored under strict deadlines, and the pressure gradually caused her to tighten. She was having trouble coming up with fresh characters, novel plot twists, and strong words to brighten her prose. At times, her ability to write shut down completely. In search of anything to cure her writer's block, Zoe joined a Buddhist meditation group where she began to sit on a regular basis, practicing "one-pointed" meditation (meaning "with a single focus"), in which she tuned out all extraneous mental clutter. In a matter of weeks, Zoe was not only more relaxed, she'd learned to witness rather than succumb to the negative thoughts that hounded her as she struggled to write. Meditation did not stop her from experiencing doubt and fear, but she was no longer controlled by these mind-states. She overcame her writer's block and recently told me she feels her writing has become more fluid and insightful since she started practicing Buddhist meditation.

Relaxation techniques can help us to develop what psychologist Mihaly Csikszentmihalyi calls "flow," that state we enter when we allow the energy behind our creative ideas to gather and move, unimpeded, toward full expression in some artistic, vocational, or recreational endeavor. Whenever we are blocked in our aesthetic expression, no matter what the cause, we can restore flow by practicing any form of relaxation that (a) reduces our anxiety and, hence, softens the ground of the creative mind; (b) allows us to witness rather than be victimized by negative or critical thoughts; and (c) helps us to connect with our unconscious or preconscious creative impulses—the free play of ideas, images, and sensations that emerge from parts of the mind we usually repress or ignore.

Meditation is not only something we do during leisure time. It is something we do so we can truly *enjoy* our leisure time. If we carry our tensions and worries with us on the "playing field," we can't play. Have you ever tried to enjoy yourself on vacation when saddled with severe financial troubles or a serious health concern about a loved one? We need to learn the skill of setting aside the troubled mind as we proceed with the important business of play, and meditation helps us do that. With practice, we discover that time and nature move forward as we sit in stillness. We can temporarily suspend our worries and our problems won't get worse. "Sit quietly, doing nothing," says the Zen Master. "Spring comes and the grass grows of itself."

Guided Imagery for Creative Living

Among the most powerful relaxation-based approaches to creativity and leisure is guided imagery. Rachel Naomi Remen, M.D., author of *Kitchen Table Wisdom*, has called imagery the "language of the unconscious," and for many women it is a portal to their innermost creative selves. You can practice breath-based relaxation followed by an imagery exercise in which you see yourself in a place you associate with peace of mind. This practice alone may help to free your creativity.

But another, more targeted, exercise is specifically designed to rouse creativity from its hiding places. Taught to me by my colleague Ann Webster, it is a guided imagery technique for creative living. Here is the simple method:

- Find a comfortable place to sit or lie, and take several slow, deep, abdominal breaths.
- To the best of your ability, clear your mind of intrusive thoughts. Take a few moments, and if any thoughts float through your consciousness, note them and then let them go. Let any nagging thoughts go with your exhalations.
- Picture yourself three months from now. Ask yourself, Where do I want to be with regard to my creativity? What would I like to be doing that best expresses my aesthetic self and uses my talents? Conjure clear pictures of yourself creating.
- Repeat this practice, this time focusing on images of yourself in leisure, enjoying yourself at play in any setting or activity that yields optimal joy.

Use this practice both to stretch your imagination and to develop new outlets for creativity and leisure. This method is also applicable to virtually any aspect of life—health, relationships, career, and spirituality. But it is particularly powerful with regard to creativity and play. Several years before I gave birth to my daughter, I observed a group led by Ann Webster, who was leading this imagery exercise. I moved from one focus to the next—health, relationships, creativity—and when we came to play, my focus suddenly settled on a mind-picture of myself with a dog. The image was so strong—I experienced such sheer joy playing with this fictional dog—that I told my husband, and together we decided to get a dog. It happened that a friend of Ann Webster's had two wonderful basset hounds, and we got in touch with their breeder. Lo and behold, the breeder told us that the dog was pregnant, and shortly therafter we picked out the eight-week-old puppy who was the liveliest of the litter. Lucy the basset hound is now a beloved member of our family.

What was most interesting to me about the imagery exercise was the fact that I had never before desired a dog—the thought had never even crossed my mind. Whether the desire was latent, or whether the desire was literally conceived during visualization, the process enabled me to open a door to a new realm of joyful relationship.

If you have any trouble with this exercise—if nothing intriguing comes to mind—you might try consciously to narrow the possibilities. For example, focus on a dream you've always had, and, if need be, excavate childhood memories to find one. Perhaps you always wanted to take piano lessons and your parents couldn't afford them, or you loved painting but never got any support from your family for your artistic passions. You may have buried these creative dreams so firmly under the sediment of years of self-denial that you've forgotten them . . . but they can be revived. The same principle applies to leisure. If you've always wanted to ride a Harley-Davidson, bungee jump, surf a wild wave, swim in a cool mountain quarry, reread Louisa May Alcott's *Little Women*, play hopscotch, or jump rope, decide that it's time to seize the opportunity.

When we're under continual stress, we stop knowing what we want. Our desires, feelings, and creative urges get lost under a cloud as we simply try to get by. Imagery for creative living allows you to clear your mind, to make room for images of yourself as creator—images that you find exciting and meaningful—and then enact them in real life. In the words of Henry David Thoreau, "Go confidently in the direction of your dreams! Live the life you've imagined."

The Healing Power of Pampering: An Approach to Leisure

You can turn your relaxation practice into a pampering ritual that restores energy and spirit after your proverbial hard day's night. A hot bath, full-body massage, or facial are genuinely relaxing and self-nurturing when you enjoy them mindfully, with senses fully open and engaged in the present. These activities are ways of integrating relaxation practice and leisure to yield the most bang for your temporal buck. We all complain that we have too little time for ourselves, too little time to relax—so we need to make the most of the time we do have.

Here's another way to look at leisure time: as an opportunity to let someone else participate in your relaxation ritual. When you get a massage from a caring and skilled bodyworker, when you receive a facial from a cosmetician with dexterous hands, when you let a reflexologist knead and press points in your feet, you invite another person to help you achieve levels of letting go you could not elicit on your own. Touch is also communication, and therapeutic forms of touch have been proven to change physiology—lowering blood pressure and heart rate while boosting certain immune functions. Psychiatrist Gail Ironson of the University of Miami has shown that a group of HIV-positive patients who received regular full-body massage experienced increases in the activity of their body's natural killer cells. Body-based treatments, which we often think of as mere indulgences, may actually be sound medicine.

So have regular pedicures, manicures, facials, acupressure treatments, shiatsu sessions, Swedish massages, and herbal wraps. If you can afford to, when you're most burned out, consider going off to a health spa for a few days of body-based relaxation and rejuvenation. But if you don't have the time or the funds, build spa-like treatments into your life by committing yourself to body-nurturing therapies on a regular basis.

Here's a brief list of additional, and less expensive, ways to pamper yourself that are also bona fide forms of relaxation:

- Lie quietly in a hammock or lounge chair until you feel fully refreshed.
- Take a bath with your favorite bubble bath or scented oils, and light candles at bathtub's edge. The oils can turn your bath into a form of aromatherapy, so select scents that induce the most comforting sensations and memories.
- Mindfully enjoy a hot bowl of chicken or fresh vegetable soup.
- Give yourself unconditional permission to take a late-afternoon nap whenever you experience tell-tale symptoms of burn-out—fatigue, headache, or loss of concentration.
- Ask your spouse, partner, or friend to rub down your back with scented oil.
- Rent a video of your favorite stand-up comedian.
- Give *yourself* a massage, working tiger balm into your forehead, upper chest, the thick band of muscles connecting neck and shoulders, arms, abdomen, and thighs.
- Select a favorite herbal tea. Pour the hot water into your mug mindfully, and sip the tea slowly, with awareness of the taste and

feel of the tea as it warms your throat and stomach. Tune out extraneous thoughts and focus solely on the successive, graceful movements and moments that comprise the simple act of drinking tea.

One sure route to relaxation deserves special mention—music. Depending on our personal tastes and memory banks, certain types of music may soothe and relax; others may elicit heart-pounding passions; still others may cause irritation or anger. But, broadly speaking, we can pick forms of music, whether classical, jazz, folk-rock, or New Age, that promote states of calmness and serenity. Rock 'n' roll is rarely calming, but it can be incredibly energizing and inspiring.

I prescribe music for women as a form of self-nurturance, with the doctorly instruction "as needed." In other words, if you need to relax, listen to music *you* find becalming; if you need inspiration, listen to music that wakes *you* up; if you need to release dark emotion, listen to selections that touch *your* grief and rage. For women in these stressful times, music can play an especially valuable role as a nonpharmaceutical tranquilizer.

FREE AT LAST: NURTURE THE PLAYFUL MIND

In the town where I live, I belong to a Bunco group. Bunco, is an extremely simple dice game, and I join a dozen other women once a month to play, schmooze, gossip, and have a few laughs. We meet at a different home each time, and I'm often a bit intimidated by my friends' beautifully decorated homes. Every room is so carefully thought out, every touch is so tasteful, from curtains and blinds to coffee tables and knick-knacks. If you detect a touch of envy in my tone, well, you're right. I'm too busy with my work and family to spend much time on interior design, and in any event, I'm not sure I have a terrific eye for home decoration.

When my turn came to host the game, I was anxious for weeks in advance. I was sure these women would come to my house, take one look around, and think: she has no creativity, she's a slob, she lacks taste, and much more. I confided my fears to my next-door neighbor, Linda, another Bunco participant who is the soul of wisdom. First, she reassured me that my home was fine (if not fabulously decorated). But then Linda said something even more important. Why should decorating a house matter so much? The other women in our group had better decorating instincts, but hadn't I been a creative designer of research projects and women's health programs? Hadn't I been creative as a book author? Of course, she was right.

My next-door neighbor had offered me the gift of cognitive restructuring. She enabled me to combat the false and unnecessary connotations of my negative thoughts about my own creativity. We are all creative in different ways.

Common negative ideas we hold about our creativity include:

I'm just not a creative person.
I'm not artistic enough.
I'm destined to fail as a painter/dancer/writer/musician/
    designer/whatever.
I have too many responsibilities to take time for creativity.
I'm too lazy to be a successful artist.
If I live out my identity as a creator, I will alienate friends and
    family.
If I try to be more creative on the job, I'll get criticized or even fired.
If I explore my artistic potential, I'll end up in the poor house.

In my experience, many people feel that they are "just not creative." If you, too, harbor this thought, I suggest you apply the four-question restructuring method to this invariably distorted idea. It is neither accurate nor fair for us to believe we lack creativity just because we may not possess extraordinary talents in the visual arts or music. The fact that I have little flair for home decoration does not mean that I lack creativity; the fact that you may not draw or write or sing is no reason to think of yourself as "uncreative," either. Broaden your view of creativity to encompass cooking, knitting, photography, printmaking, joke-telling, mimicry, doodling, floral arranging, gardening, even finger painting. As a cognitive approach, I often suggest to patients that they list hobbies or skills they never previously considered creative.

For instance, a close friend, Betsy, doesn't consider herself a professional painter or designer. But she and her husband bought a house a few years ago, and she turned certain rooms into works of art, painting her kitchen walls with elaborate, witty depictions of fruits and vegetables and her dining room with vibrant colors and calligraphy. Despite her obvious talents—Betsy is one of the most creative people I know—she doesn't identify herself as the true artist she is. Her motto, "It's only paint—I can always repaint."

The question, "Where did I get this thought," can be pivotal, since too many women have received a lifetime of negative messages about their creative worth and potential. One writer I know characterized her childhood training: "My parents' communication was, 'Be a good girl, do your homework, do what your teacher tells you, be quiet, don't be messy.' My teachers were saying pretty much the same thing: It was, 'Get the right answer,' not 'think on your own creatively.' These instructions made it hard for me later as a writer. As any kind of artist, you need to cultivate a messy mind, like a child who's free with her many colored paints. The messages I got put order and good behavior above all else . . . not the best way to fertilize the creative spirit."

Of course, "I'm destined to fail" is a greatest hit, one that takes work to overcome. Those of us plagued by fear and doubt are usually saddled with outsized expectations about what it means to be a successful creator. We believe we must be Georgia O'Keeffe, Virginia Woolf, Cecelia Bartoli, Martha Graham, Meryl Streep—or nothing. As Julia Cameron points out in her liberating book, *The Artist's Way*, "The need to be a great artist makes it hard to be an artist. The need to produce a great work of art makes it hard to produce any art at all." We must get rid of our concepts of aesthetic greatness. We can't make our own personal artistic explorations, or even get started on our own creative journeys, when we're hamstrung by impossible goals, usually rooted in unreachable standards set for us by parents and teachers.

Here are two sample restructurings of negative thoughts about creativity:

NEGATIVE THOUGHT: "I don't deserve to be artistic."
RESTRUCTURED THOUGHT: "I never felt deserving since I was brought
                       up to believe that my first and foremost
                       job was to raise a family. Not only that, I
                       was led to think that being an artist was
                       some privileged gift bestowed by God

upon certain fortunate beings, the Mozarts and Rembrandts and Ballanchines and Bernhardts of the world. Moreover, women were far less likely than men to be counted among the lucky ones. But now I see family and friends pursuing their creativity, and I recognize that we all have a right to artistic expression. I was susceptible to these attitudes because of my own low self-esteem. I have no less right to work on my painting and drawing than anyone else, and I owe it to myself to take time for my creative development."

NEGATIVE THOUGHT: "If I live out my identity as a creator, I will alienate friends and family."

RESTRUCTURED THOUGHT: "I may alienate some people, since I will be devoting more time to my art, which means less time at my job; a somewhat reduced income; and less time with my husband and friends. But should I neglect my creativity for fear of their disapproval or hurt feelings? Or, should I try my best to communicate my desires to them, letting them know that I will miss the extra time but that I need to pursue artistic expression in order to be a whole person? My husband is capable of understanding this, and friends who are genuinely loyal and loving will understand, too. I can be articulate and tenacious enough to make my needs clear and stick to my principles. In the long run, my relationships may even be strengthened, and I can sacrifice some income to pursue creative endeavors."

Leisure Without Guilt

Women should also apply the cognitive approach to hounding negative thoughts about leisure time. "Down time" is the first to go in our daily grind, and guilt over taking "too much" down time—however much that is—comes from inner voices pestering us to be constantly productive.

Guilt can be healthy. When we procrastinate for too long over a work project, guilt gives us a much-needed kick in the butt. When we're really spending too little quality time with our kids, we *ought* to feel bad about it. But most women I know are frequently saddled with excessive guilt over perceived or projected lapses that aren't lapses at all.

With regard to self-nurturing leisure time, we can learn a thing or two from men. Yes, men. In the next chapter, I'll describe the "female bonding" days I've enjoyed with a close group of women friends. But the truth is, we got the idea from our husbands, who had "male bonding" days on an annual basis. When we realized how much fun they had—how revitalizing it was for them to watch ball games and "shoot the shit"—we decided we deserved the same pleasure. Though our activities were decidedly different (hot tubs, confessional storytelling, and "chick" movie rentals), our sense of entitlement was the same. Use your male partners, friends, and family members as examples; observe how much less guilty they feel about unadulterated leisure time and decide that you're entitled to the same freedoms.

Here is an unfortunate cognitive distortion: Self-nurture is hedonism! (Dictionary definition of hedonism: "Devotion to pleasure and self-gratification as a way of life.") Women bitten by the productivity bug believe that taking time for self-nurturing leisure is no different from the unrestrained pursuit of personal pleasure at the expense of anything and everything else in their lives. Hogwash! Women must start from the premise that in our frenzied world we need and deserve time to recharge. We must also acknowledge our right to pleasure—emotional, intellectual, creative, physical, sensual—as long as pleasure is not the whole of our existence. The pursuit of pleasure can only be called hedonism when it eclipses compassion for others, and a sense of responsibility to our loved ones and communities.

Another familiar distortion? Self-nurture *is selfish*. While I know a few selfish women who disguise their narcissism as self-care, they are few and far between. Far more women deny themselves revitalizing pleasures because they believe they should be spending their time tending to others. These women tend to be self-sacrificing at their own expense, not egotistically self-involved.

In my experience, three broad categories of women are plagued by negative thoughts about leisure. The first is the career-focused single woman so deeply involved in work that she feels there can be no time for play. The second is the full-time mother deeply engaged in child-rearing. The third is the working mother trying to juggle everything at once. All three entertain somewhat different yet equally corrosive ideas about leisure, and all three can restructure these beliefs. Here are typical negative thoughts and sample restructurings:

SINGLE WORKING WOMAN: "If I take too much time to chill out, I'll never get my work done and fully succeed in my career."

RESTRUCTURING: "If I don't get enough down time, I will eventually succumb to the law of diminishing returns and burn out before my time. Also, in focusing exclusively on work, I often lose sight of other aspects of life that need tending—my body, relationships, spiritual growth, helping others, unadulterated play. I owe it to myself to cultivate more balance."

FULL-TIME MOTHER: "How can I take more time for leisure when it's subtracted from time with my kids?"

RESTRUCTURING: "If I don't get enough leisure time, I will find myself exhausted, inattentive, even resentful as I take care of my children. If I enlist my husband and others to take over when I need to relax, revitalize, and play, I will actually become a more present and loving mother, and my children will know and feel it. I'm going to be a better role model for my daughter/son if I can demonstrate to them that I can self-nurture. As adults, my daughter will feel entitled to nurture herself and my son will support his wife in her efforts to self-nurture."

WORKING MOTHER: "I can barely get through the day with my work and child-rearing responsibilities; there's no way I can take more time for sheer leisure without shirking obligations."

RESTRUCTURING: "Given my daily load, there are long stretches when I feel like a drudge. The only way to change that is to give myself the gift of uninterrupted time for my own pleasure and relaxation. If I really evaluate how I spend my time, the fact is, I can reshuffle priorities and schedules to find at least a half-hour each day to read the paper, take a bath, listen to great music, or get my husband to give me a massage."

THE UNCHAINED IMAGINATION: NURTURE THE EMOTIONS

Many "normal" women have trouble birthing their own creative works. Julia Cameron calls them "blocked creatives," and she offers a spate of writing exercises to help them over their perennial humps. As a psychologist I'm interested in helping women find out why they are blocked creatives. Writing is a good tool for figuring this out, and figuring this out is a powerful way to transcend your block. For instance, many women have been taught from the earliest age that it's okay to be creative in the kitchen or home but not outside. (This notion is far less prevalent than it was twenty and thirty years ago, but many of my patients still struggle with this antiquated and unfortunate lesson.) In this regard, I was lucky. My mother didn't care much about home design or whether our meals were delectable, as long as the house was clean and we were well nourished. She was, however, passionately concerned with her creative growth outside the home, and she instilled that philosophy in my sister and myself. Few women I know got this message when young, and it can take some exploration to overcome this early lack. I suggest these writing exercises:

1. Write out your thoughts and feelings about yourself as a creative person. In what ways has your creativity been expressed, and in what ways has it been blocked?

2. What messages did you get from your parents, teachers, and others about your creativity? Were your creative actions taken seriously? Praised? Belittled? Ignored? Which messages stayed with you, and which ones have you jettisoned? How do they affect you today?

3. When you think of being creative, what's the first thing that flashes into your mind? Forget what others think or what you think you should do. . . . What image seems to fulfill your vision of yourself as a creator, an artist, a whole person?

Unleashing Your Play Potential

Emotional factors can prevent us from leisurely play, just as they block us from creative expression. When it comes to early training in productivity, I had a rather complex background. My mother wanted her daughters to succeed, and we always got her wholehearted support for our efforts to build professional lives. But she also espoused self-nurture and leisurely play. I remember her doing crossword puzzles no matter how cluttered the house was. By contrast, my father was an exceptionally diligent professor who'd never relax until all his work was completed. Given these role models, I have spent virtually my entire life swinging back and forth between extremes of all work (my father's example) and all play (my mother's influence).

Early on, I tended to embrace the priority of hard work over leisure. By high school, I was more interested in boys and volunteering than schoolwork. In college, I swung back toward work, becoming obsessed with good grades. After graduate school, I went through a period, as a single woman with extra time, of almost overindulgent self-nurturance. As my professional life solidified, I reverted back to my college-era preoccupation with achievement. Since the birth of my daughter several years ago, my work/family time crunch has challenged my commitment to self-nurture. It has been a particular struggle for me to balance my needs and my daughter's needs. I still must fend off the inner voice berating me whenever I choose time for myself when my work or my daughter waits in the wings.

Why are we so prone to self-denial? I have a theory, which is based on the tenets of child development. Prior to the age of five or six, children lack the ego development to understand that their parents (and anyone else, for that matter) have valid needs. Young children view the world strictly through the lens of their emotional desires and physical urgencies. During this early phase, parents' attempts to explain their needs ("Honey, your father and I are going to a movie; your grandmother will take care of you till we get home") may be met with confusion, sorrow, or anger. I don't call this "narcissism." Rather, children under five simply don't have the brain development to comprehend parental needs and autonomy.

Certainly, some women had neglectful parents who always put their own needs ahead of their children. If the experience was traumatic, and we harbored a deep-seated resentment, we might have learned to equate a healthy sense of self-nurture with selfishness. Years later, the child within us remains bewildered by or angry at anyone who appears to put their needs over those of a family member or child and we apply this same standard to ourselves. We constantly hound ourselves with the question, "How dare I . . ." or "How dare she . . . ?"

Once in a blue moon, when I tell my three-year-old daughter, Sarah, that I want to read the newspaper for a few minutes rather than play with her, she does everything she can to sabotage me. I remain patient, letting her know that I am there for her when she needs me, but that Mommy needs a few moments for herself.

Once we understand the emotional basis for our unwillingness to grant ourselves time for pleasure, we can take the paradoxical step of tending seriously to the business of play. We can recognize that our health and well-being depend on built-in blocks of time for activities with only one purpose: to bring us joy. One way to accomplish this is the **Time Pie**.

The Time Pie

The time-pie exercise, taught to me by my colleague Ann Webster, will help you accomplish two goals at once: to identify activities that yield emotions of pure joy and serenity, and to find time for them on a regular basis.

Draw a circle on a piece of paper, and create a pie chart of your typical twenty-four-hour day. If you usually sleep eight hours each night, draw a slice that represents one-third of the pie. Then draw a slice that represents the number of hours you devote to work each day. Next, figure out approximately how much time you spend on other activities: commuting, cooking and eating meals, shopping, caretaking, making love, watching TV, showering, doing chores, etc. Write the activity in each slice until your whole pie (24-hour day) consists of large slices and small slivers of time. Here is a sample time pie:

Sample Time Pie

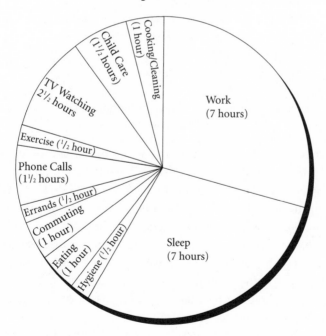

Now put aside your time pie. On another piece of paper, write down the numbers 1 through 20 in a vertical column. As quickly as you can—without lengthy deliberation—list twenty things that bring you joy and serenity. Here is a sample list from one of my patients:

1. Nature walks
2. Hanging out in the library
3. Listening to old Motown records
4. Spending time with my favorite niece and nephew
5. Making love with my husband
6. Watching movies from the 1940s
7. Shopping for shoes
8. Daydreaming
9. Reading books on spirituality and health
10. Going to comedy clubs
11. Practicing yoga
12. Talking on the phone with faraway friends
13. Having lunch with my sister
14. Listening to poetry readings or great novels on tape
15. Long country walks in mild, sunny weather
16. Cooking and enjoying an exotic meal
17. Going out dancing with friends
18. Surfing the net
19. Laughing with my husband while lying in bed
20. Running four miles around the park

Now compare your list of twenty with your time pie. How much time is indicated on the pie for any of the activities listed? Of course, there may be pastimes on your list that you wouldn't do that frequently, like going to a comedy club. But others, like daydreaming or reading, might ideally be part of a typical day. Do these activities show up on our time pie? Many women who follow this exercise discover that there is *no* time on their pie for any of the twenty items. Others count the time spent on purely joyful activity in minutes rather than hours. This can be a shocking revelation, one that motivates some women to radically transform the way they spend their time.

Next, redraw your time pie to include a few slices of time for at least some of your joyful activities. Start with your old pie and make whatever changes necessary—cutting certain sections down or out—to create space for the most important items on your list. Don't let this become an exercise in pure fantasy; be as realistic as possible. And be tough-minded: if you watch too many sitcoms or spend hours in gabfests on the phone, cut back and use the extra time for reading, yoga, making love, walks in the park—whatever brings you the most peace of mind and happiness.

Redrawn Time Pie

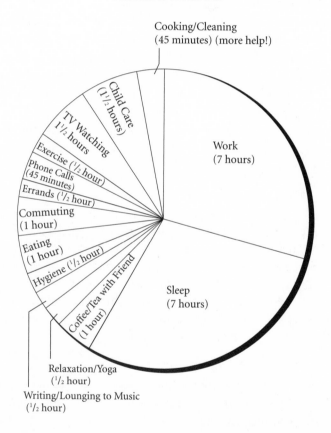

Cooking/Cleaning
(45 minutes) (more help!)

Child Care
(1½ hours)

TV Watching
1½ hours

Exercise (½ hour)

Phone Calls
(45 minutes)

Errands (½ hour)

Commuting
(1 hour)

Eating
(1 hour)

Hygiene (½ hour)

Coffee/Tea with Friend
(1 hour)

Work
(7 hours)

Sleep
(7 hours)

Relaxation/Yoga
(½ hour)

Writing/Lounging to Music
(½ hour)

NOTE: Fifteen minutes borrowed from cooking and cleaning (more help from family!), along with one less hour of watching television and 45 minutes less phone chatting yields two extra hours per day—time for relaxation/yoga, writing or lounging to music, or coffee or tea with a friend.

The time pie is merely a tool to help you identify chunks of time spent in unrewarding or self-sacrificing activities, then redirect them toward soul-nourishing activities that replenish your energies and revive your spirit.

ACTS OF CREATION, DAYS OF REST:
NURTURE THE SELF/SPIRIT

Elizabeth, the patient I spoke about in chapter 4, is a seventy-two-year-old woman with non-Hodgkin's lymphoma. She had been an interior decorator, and she and her husband, Marvin, ran a studio specializing in wall coverings and fabrics. Prior to her diagnosis a few years ago, Elizabeth and Marvin closed up shop, largely because she wanted to spend more time with her grandchildren. Elizabeth remained active after retirement, volunteering to lead schoolchildren in tours of art museums. But her diagnosis motivated her to more fully investigate her creative desires, and further, to fill her days with richly pleasurable activity.

First, Elizabeth applied self-nurturing wisdom during months of intensive chemotherapy:

> I actually enjoyed this period in bed, because I confronted myself with the question, "If I'm going to lie here, what am I going to do with my time?" And I got such pleasure hearing classical music, reading, and listening to books on tape. When I was well enough to sit on our porch and look out at nature and listen to the birds, I savored every second. Maybe it's my age and maturity, but I never had this feeling that I should be doing this or doing that. I gave myself permission to lie there and basically nourish myself with works of art.

Here's a brief version of Elizabeth's menu during her treatment and convalescence: playing Beethoven and Mozart CDs; reading Hemingway and other great American and European novelists; listening to books on audiotape, including Tolstoy's *Anna Karenina* and Austen's *Pride and Prejudice*; and listening to National Public Radio talk shows. Her voracious appetite for learning and culture served her well—Elizabeth's immersion in music and books fed her spiritual life, buttressing her sense of meaning and purpose as she lay in bed hoping for a full recovery.

As her energy rebounded, Elizabeth became more active in her creative and leisurely pursuits. She embarked on various home renovation projects. "I love fixing and doing and creating in my environment. I enjoy every minute and every inch of it." She joined a gardening club and two reading clubs, took herself to movie matinees, went on antiquing excursions, attended ballet and opera concerts. She and Marvin joined a *havurah,* immersing themselves in Jewish learning, culture, and prayer. Elizabeth is now actively seeking a role as a volunteer to help people with serious illness navigate their way through the medical system.

"We're not here very long," explained Elizabeth. "I thank God I have the strength to take advantage of whatever time I have."

In her encounter with illness, Elizabeth rediscovered her sense of deservedness, filling her days with engaging, entertaining, and emotionally uplifting pursuits. Now, Elizabeth is in complete remission from lymphoma. She is a shining example of this basic lesson in self-care: We nurture the spirit within the self when we embark on the creative quest, find joy in simple pleasures, or just let ourselves wind down to a sweet stillness.

The Spirit of Creativity

Many writers and artists have described the creative endeavor as an act of faith, and creative inspiration as a spark of the divine. You need only contemplate memories of your own moments of creative vision to recognize that something unexplainable happens—ideas, melodies, insights, or images come spontaneously, without warning, from a part of your mind or soul that you cannot fully fathom. Whether you believe the source is the unconscious, the unfettered imagination, spiritual "energy," or a personal God, you realize that you've become, however briefly, a vehicle for a creative force.

You must safeguard that creative spirit. Julia Cameron echoes my beliefs in *The Artist's Way:* "The essential element in nurturing our creativity lies in nurturing ourselves. Through self-nurturance we nurture our inner connection to the Great Creator. Through this connection our creativity will unfold. Paths will appear for us. We need to trust the Great Creator and move out in faith."

Spirit moves through us during creative inspiration, but we should not sit around waiting to be thunderstruck by a divine spark. Rather, we must deliberately make space for opportunities to be creative, doing the playful work involved—composing poems, drafting sketches, practicing musical instruments, perfecting dance steps, etc. The creative process is just that—a process involving elements of craft, technique, learning, and imaginative play. Through it all, we undergo periods of boredom, engagement, distraction, ecstasy, dreaminess, anxiety, and, yes, sudden bursts of enlightenment. If we stick with the process, sooner or later we'll be rewarded with those bursts. But the way to safeguard our creative spirit is *to engage in the process,* with all its fallow periods.

Sometimes, creativity is a route to corners of the soul we didn't know existed. "It is indeed from the experience of beauty and happiness, from the occasional harmony between our nature and our environment, that we draw our conception of the divine life," wrote philosopher George Santayana. Artistic creation can lead us to that experience of beauty and harmony from which "we draw our conception of the divine life."

At various stressful times in my life, I've found immense peace of mind in creative expression. I recall the year I wrote my doctoral dissertation, a time of near-constant pressure. I bought myself a box of watercolors and felt markers, and spent much of my spare time creating abstract designs and filling in picture books. I'm not sure if I ever broke through to a creative epiphany, but I felt a serenity and wholeness that contrasted with my dissertation-induced frenzy. Nine years ago, I was overloaded with work, house hunting, and wedding plans. I couldn't relax, so I decided to take an evening pottery course. I learned how to use the electric wheel. For two hours, I'd lose myself—and my troubles—in the whirring pottery wheel, which had an almost hypnotic effect. The total focus required—a single slip and your pot is ruined—led me into a state of mindfulness.

Perhaps you are stymied about how best to cultivate the spirit of creativity in your own life. Maybe you've tried drawing, painting, or writing and none of them grab you, or you don't feel you have sufficient talents in those areas to merit spending time on them. Here, then, is a short list of creative pursuits I have compiled from the experience of patients, friends, and acquaintances. These are women who march to their own beat, finding joy, tranquility, freedom, and self-transcendence in a wide range of artistic endeavors:

- **Gardening:** Not usually credited as a creative activity, but true gardeners know better. Many women find peace in the garden, partly because they commune with the earth, partly because they lose themselves in the visual splendor of their flowers and plants. But gardening is an authentic act of creation: the gardener's choice of flowers, placement, landscaping, and other touches are little different from the choices of painters and architects.

- **Movement:** How many of us have the talent to be a professional dancer? Does that mean we can't find artistic expression in movement or dance? Surely not. Dance and movement classes give you the opportunity to let your body speak for you and to you, to release energies that are as creative as any verbal or visual medium would allow.
- **Karaoke:** In the same spirit, we can't all be rock stars or pop icons, but we can sing out our hearts with the guidance of our favorite tracks playing on stereos at homes or in karaoke clubs. Admittedly an activity on the border of creativity and leisure, it still gives us a chance for vocal expression in a thoroughly joyful context.
- **Poetry:** I know women who have not written a word since college, and others who've only written technical papers, nonfiction, or business briefs, who discovered another part of their brains by writing poetry. In some alchemical way, the form lends itself to deep expression of feeling; poetry asks us to bypass the left-brain intellectual mind and reach down into the soul of experience.
- **Musical Instruments:** Pick up an instrument you loved and lost, or one you never tried at all. Electric or acoustic guitar, piano, clarinet, harmonica, violin, cello, bass, drums—whatever strikes a chord with you, as it were. If you can devote time to practice and eventual technical excellence, great. If not, proceed in a spirit of play and tune out critical voices: your goal is musical expression and pleasure, not musical stardom.
- **Acting:** Take an acting class! I know many women who have found acting to be an enormously liberating and creatively challenging endeavor. Forget Streep, Sarandon, and Lange: explore your own emotional and imaginative resources.

The Spirit of Leisure

It may seem like a trivial subject, but it's not trivial at all. A spiritual life may depend on how we spend our leisure time.

I split leisure into two broad categories: doing something and doing nothing. There is an art to both. In the "doing" category, we can engage in activities that are dulling, that do not lead to greater serenity, pleasure, insight, or genuine fun. (I'm thinking of excessive TV watching, video game playing, net surfing, and phone gabbing.) But there are active forms of leisure that are truly revitalizing (more shortly). There are also ways to do absolutely nothing that evoke profound inner peace. As Jon Kabat-Zinn has said, "Don't just do something, sit there." Just sitting there—or bathing, lounging, or lying there—is restorative when practiced in the spirit of self-nurture.

What are revitalizing forms of active leisure? Activities that generate inner peace, or those that rouse a sense of fun rooted in our childlike spontaneity. Find opportunities such as these:

- **Bookstore Lounging:** Go to one of those roomy bookstores with plush chairs and spend hours browsing, skimming, and reading.
- **Classical Concerts:** Whether or not you're a classical music fan, try taking yourself to hear a symphony orchestra or chamber music concert. You may experience a musical revelation.
- **Eat Childhood Foods:** Some of us suffer from continual dietary restriction—fears of fat and sugar so excessive that we avoid tasty foods like the plague or punish ourselves for a single indulgence. Low-fat and -sugar diets are health-promoting, but if guilt and shame characterize your relationship with food, you should occasionally indulge your desire for forbidden childhood delights—an ice-cream sundae, piece of birthday cake, fruit pie, or chocolate pudding with whipped cream. Shut out guilt before, during, and afterward.
- **Live Theater:** If you're like me, you rarely find the time or take the opportunity to see a play or musical show. Live theater is a wonderful antidote to our TV and movie culture. We get to commune with live actors, whose performance in the here and now can't be predicted, whose energy and sweat and passion are palpable to us.
- **Soul-Nourishing Celluloid:** Rent movies that have meant something to you in the past—films that represented an emotional or spiritual watershed at some time during your life, whether childhood, adolescence, or adulthood. I know women who feel that their lives were changed forever, for the better, by certain movies. Watch these films and reawaken the primal feelings and insights they first stimulated.

- **Amusement Park:** Take yourself and your partner, with or without kids, to an amusement park, and let yourself go. If there is a park you went to as a child and haven't been there in decades, all the better.
- **Museums and Galleries:** Take yourself on what Julia Cameron calls an "artist's date" to an art museum or gallery. Most of us tend to neglect the pantheons of art in our midst. If you live in or near a big city, explore the art museums and galleries in a spirit of mindfulness, observing the paintings, drawings, and sculpture with a wide-open mind.

We can also creatively use leisure time to heal ourselves from psychological distress, which can also be good for our health. I recently came across a wonderful collection of cards written by Lynn Gordon, "52 Silly Things to Do When You Are Blue," which reflects my own approach to healing depression through self-nurturing leisure. Here are several of Gordon's inventive suggestions, with a few of her notes, adapted from her cards:

- **Go Fly a Kite:** When was the last time you indulged in a childhood—okay, maybe not even your own childhood—activity like flying a kite or going roller skating?
- **Life History:** Write a list of fifty good things that have happened in your life, from finding your lost turtle in the second grade to the name of the person who first said you had a beautiful smile.
- **Feed the Birds:** Dig out those dried-out English muffins or the loaf of eighteen-grain bread that never got eaten, and head to a park. Find a picturesque bench and feed the squirrels or birds.
- **Mystery Adventure:** Hop on public transportation and spontaneously go somewhere you've never been but have always wanted to visit. Pretend you are a travel writer covering a new adventure.
- **Clean a Closet:** Clean out a closet or empty that junk-filled kitchen drawer. Get rid of the excess clothes and clap-trap you've been living with by donating it all to a favorite community thrift shop.
- **Favorite Music Mix:** Sort through all your albums, cassettes, or CDs and make a tape of your favorite music. You could make one easy-listening tape and one hard-core dance-till-you-drop tape.

- **Make an Album:** Make a photo album of your friends and loved ones. Track down photos you don't have and take pictures of friends near you. This is a good thing to have around to remind yourself of what's really important and who loves you.

I've offered you options for active leisure, but just as important are the "do nothing" options. Many of them fall under the relaxation category: meditation, massage, body work, and other ways to achieve deep rest by sitting or lying still. One purpose of these methods is to recover from the burnout of overscheduling and overdoing. Ask yourself: What do I need to rebound from severe stress and exhaustion? What does my mind need? What does my body need? What does my spirit need? These are simple questions, but they should be asked and answered with the greatest possible truthfulness and clarity.

The Personal Retreat

I was inspired by a story on *Oprah* of a woman who went on a personal retreat. She'd been burned out by an overscheduled lifestyle, and she healed her distress and fatigue by taking an entire month at home, in solitude, to tend to her spirit. The following is a blueprint for your own personal retreat.

Imagine the experience of an extravagant health spa without the extravagant bill. If you can, stay home by yourself for one week. If you can't take a week off from work, give yourself a week or two of retreat while remaining at work—filling your evenings and weekends with quiet reflection and self-nurturance. Ask your husband to free you up by taking charge of child care. Use the time for meditation; contemplation; gentle exercise; mindful walks in nature; hot baths and other forms of hydrotherapy; aromatherapy; journaling; recording your dreams and creative visions; long naps; and rituals of prayer and spiritual observance. Cut out TV, magazines, and newspapers—only read material that is spiritually enlivening. Okay, so you won't have a personal cook or strong-handed body workers at the ready. But you will have the total freedom to tend to mind, body, and soul as you wish, with no external pressures or people around to please.

Another way to manage if you have children is to find a friend with children who'll take your kids for one weekend while you go on "retreat." Then you can take her kids the following weekend. If there are so many children involved that the idea seems burdensome, try this for just one Saturday. Even a single day of such pure self-nurturing relaxation can yield big dividends. You can "invite" your husband to take that weekend trip with the buddies he'd been craving, or to relocate at a relative's house, so you can give yourself the gift of solitude. It's a radical idea, but one you can arrange as long as you stick with your convictions.

In many respects, self-nurturing leisure is also about time—namely, the maximal use of time for our emotional and spiritual well-being. Unfortunately, many of today's time-management tomes are oriented toward the better use of time for maximal productivity. I believe that a self-nurturing approach to time will actually help some of us become more productive by boosting our energy levels and healing burnout, but these are side benefits. We must embrace the use of time for creativity and leisure because it is good for the body and good for the soul. I recently came upon this eloquent commentary by Mary C. Morrison in her book *Let Evening Come: Reflections on Aging*:

> Where has time gone? When I was growing up, seventy years ago, there was plenty of time, the best sort of time. Time to goof off, to do nothing, and simply grow. Even in my children's growing up days they had that kind of time, at least in the summers, to lie in hammocks and read and think and just grow. The need to grow doesn't stop, even in old age; and I think I do some of my best growing when I'm lying in bed in the morning, slowly getting my eyes open. I wonder if the interest in meditation these days is not perhaps an attempt to find this lost and legendary treasure, time. Of course in the Eastern cultures, it is usually billed as timelessness; but for us Westerners, I think it is really time that we are looking for. I wonder if it vanished when digital watches came in, presenting, as they do, one isolated second vanishing into another endlessly—in contrast to clock faces, which show time visually as a waiting space. I am coming to have a real sense of time as the fourth dimension, a lost aspect of the space in which a truly human life is lived.

7

FRIENDS AND SIBLINGS:

SOCIAL SUPPORT IN ACTION

Oh, the comfort, the inexpressible comfort of feeling safe with a person, having neither to weigh thoughts nor measure words, but pouring them all out, just as they are, chaff and grain together, certain that a faithful hand will take and sift them, keep what is worth keeping and with a breath of kindness blow the rest away.

—Dinah Maria Mulock Clark

I HAVE SEVERAL FRIENDS from high school—three women and one man—with whom I've been fortunate to stay close to over the years. All four friends are married and have children, and my husband, Dave, and I usually get together with these couples every month or so. No particular reason is needed for us to make a date, though we do traditionally gather on special occasions—a summer pool party, New Year's Eve, and the Super Bowl. Three years ago, while I was away on a business trip, Dave invited the men over to our house for a male-bonding day of sports watching, beer drinking, and backyard basketball. They had such an enjoyable time that they decided to make it an annual event. The next yearly male-bonding gathering led the women in our group to say to our husbands and ourselves, "Fair is fair. If we are going to watch the kids all day so you can male bond, we need our own female-bonding day."

Last year, the men had their day while the five women took the kids, and a month later, we had our day together while the men assumed child-care duties. Predictably, the men stuck to their sports-oriented routine, and perhaps just as predictably, the women chose a different way to connect. We gathered at one of our homes where we watched two "chick" movies, and afterward sat in our friend's hot tub and sipped strawberry daiquiris.

As we sipped our drinks in the hot tub, we poured out our hearts. My father had just died, and I talked about my relationship with him and the impact of his death. That prompted one friend to speak of her own father's death. We discovered that both of us had experienced major shifts in our relationships with our mothers since our fathers had died, and it was reassuring to share our similar experiences. We each told our stories and shed some tears, any inhibitions having been washed away by our sense of closeness, not to mention the hot bubbling water and the alcohol.

Except perhaps for the very generous amounts of chips and chocolate we consumed, we regretted nothing that went on that day. It was sheer pleasure to spend those hours with such wonderful friends.

How often do women have this sort of opportunity? Today's world seems constructed in such a way that we are rarely so fortunate. We need close friendships and sibling relationships as surely as we need the nourishment of nutritious food, yet there are times when we barely can schedule a lunch date with just one friend.

I consider this a terrible bind, since it's the height of self-nurture to cultivate time with friends and siblings. When I was in college, I read Marilyn French's classic novel, *The Women's Room*, which chronicled the development of a group of women from prefeminist days through the feminist movement of the late sixties and early seventies. At the novel's outset, the protagonist, Mira Ward, is introduced as a young mother who typifies 1950s womanhood. She's at home with her young children, and her husband's expectations are crystal clear: She is to have the house spotlessly clean, the kids bathed and dressed, and food on the table by six o'clock sharp. French dramatizes the frustrations of Mira and her female friends with this sort of personal and cultural confinement, which comes to a head with Mira's divorce and the sweeping social changes wrought by feminism.

What fascinated me was how French made it seem like the big social changes were hatched by close female cohorts caught together in the same stultifying trap. They were stuck in the women's room, but they had each another. Mira and her friends, true to the lives of most married women in this country prior to the late sixties, met everyday to drink coffee and talk about their lives while their kids played together. They exchanged grievances and hopes, desperations and dreams. On a grand scale, the bonds they forged transformed our society. Yet as the sixties gave way to the seventies, the positive social changes also began to shred the very fabric of the female friendships that helped bring about these changes.

How so? As women increasingly began to develop their potential—entering colleges, pursuing graduate-level educations, and joining the work world before settling down with family—something was lost. I believe that few women have the same close ties at work that women in earlier times had with their mothers, sisters, cousins, and neighbors. While they are often fulfilled in their careers, they still feel isolated because their work friendships don't always have the closeness and intensity of those forged in the homes and neighborhoods of the past. I certainly know exceptions, but frequently the intense relationships formed on the job don't extend beyond the temporal boundaries of nine to five. And in some workplaces, where women are encouraged to compete against one another for raises, promotions, or better titles, there's little opportunity even to develop a sense of camaraderie and cooperation.

This subtle fraying of female bonds has bred a strangely unfeminist phenomenon: women looking to men to meet all their needs. In the old days, women's intellectual and creative needs were not met but their emotional needs often were—by other women in the home and community. More recently, working women have so little down time—and so few strong ties with fellow workers—that they turn to their male partners to take up most of the slack. This puts too much pressure on partnerships, and women are often left hungry for the companionship of female confidantes.

I'm certainly not wishing for a return to the 1950s, but I believe it is supremely self-nurturing for women to reconstruct the kind of friendships—whether with friends, or with brothers and sisters—that our mothers and grandmothers had in abundance. This chapter is devoted to specific ways you can nurture your friendships and sibling relationships. I will focus more on female friendships and sisters, simply because, for most women, they are a greater source of sustenance. Of course, I also know women who get much succor from male friends and brothers. But I have no doubt that women are uniquely empathic toward other women.

Health Benefits of the Social Safety Net

Before offering you techniques for nurturing yourself in the context of friendships and sibling relationships, you may be surprised to learn about the extraordinary health benefits of a strong social safety net. This "net" is certainly woven together by family ties, but studies suggest that friendships and strong-knit communities are essential components.

A prime example is the small hamlet of Roseto, an Italian-American town in the foothills of eastern Pennsylvania. Roseto was settled in 1882 by immigrants from an Italian village of the same name, and the settlers re-created and retained in Pennsylvania the cultural and social traditions of their European hometown. A group of researchers has studied inhabitants of Roseto for nearly four decades, and their findings give us a glimpse of how old-style community ties generate not only warmth and good will, but resistance to disease as well. When Stewart Wolf and John G. Bruhn began their research, they found that Roseto's death rate from heart attacks was significantly lower than three neighboring communities and the country as a whole. Wolf and Bruhn ruled out other explanations, such as a better diet. Indeed, the inhabitants of Roseto consumed more animal fats high in cholesterol than their neighbors and other Americans.

What Rosetans had in abundance, however, was familial and community closeness characterized by three-generation households, intraethnic marriages, devoted church-going, membership in social groups, and an overall neighborliness. By contrast, the nearby towns with higher mortality rates did not have the same close-knit community ties.

During the 1960s, the social fabric of Roseto began to fray, and the resulting effects on the health and well-being of Rosetans have fascinating ramifications. Wolf and Bruhn observed trends of "Americanization," in which citizens of the town began to move away, marry outside the clan, pursue material goals, and abandon cultural and religious customs. With these trends came a concomitant rise in heart disease deaths. Today, the mortality rates in Roseto more closely resemble those of neighboring towns and the country as a whole. Surprisingly, the death rate has risen in Roseto despite the fact that the town's inhabitants are eating less fatty and cholesterol-rich foods! The risks associated with disintegrating social networks may be even greater than those associated with such proven dangers as a high-fat diet.

A few years ago, we spoke with a long-surviving member of the Roseto community, sixty-nine-year-old Mamie Ciliberti. Mamie remembers how it used to be. "My parents were not materialistic. What was important to them was family, hard work, being together with friends, and good times. . . . My mom and dad lived with us, and helped raise the children. We all got along." The "we" was a large group—Mamie and her husband, James, had seven children. "My kids say it today: 'We're so fortunate to have had Grandmom and Grandpop.' "

Mamie wistfully recalled how Rosetans would stroll down Garibaldi Avenue, the town's main street. "Folks would walk by and greet friends who sat on porches lining the street. That's how they would socialize. Today, people don't walk anymore—except maybe by themselves in the morning to get exercise." Garibaldi Avenue used to be lined with the small shops that made it the center of social activity. "There was a butcher shop, a drugstore, a bakery, a bank, and an shoemaker," says Mamie. "But there are no stores down there anymore. Now, everyone drives to another part of town to the IGA supermarket."

The Roseto research provides compelling evidence that such alterations in the social fabric of communities can compromise our health. Here are some other key pieces of evidence, including long-term population-based studies, that prove the health-promoting value of strong social ties:

- The Alameda County Study: Lisa Berkman and Leonard Syme led a study of almost 7,000 men and women in Alameda County, California. Over the nine-year follow-up period, people who lacked strong community and social ties were 1.9 to 3.1 times more likely to die. The risk associated with inadequate social support was independent of other risk factors, including age, smoking, socioeconomic status, overeating, insufficient exercise, and health status at the study's outset.
- The Finland Study: Over 13,000 people were tracked for between five and nine years. Those who were socially isolated had a two- to threefold increased risk of death compared with those who had ample social connections and a sense of community. The researchers found that this statistical relationship held strong after controlling for age, smoking, cholesterol, and blood pressure.

- The Swedish Studies: More than 17,000 men and women were followed for six years. Those who reported being most isolated and lonely were nearly four times more likely to die prematurely than those with adequate social networks. The researchers left no stone unturned in their search for alternative explanations: age, sex, smoking, educational status, exercise habits, and preexisting diseases. But no other factor explained the relationship between social isolation and early death.

- Dr. James House's Review: In 1990, epidemiologist James House of the University of Michigan published a landmark paper in which he reviewed a half-dozen studies, including several mentioned above, with a total of more than 22,000 men and women. He demonstrated that people without strong networks of social support were two to four times more likely to die than those with rich, substantial networks.

- Heart Disease and Social Support: Redford Williams, M.D., of Duke University tracked almost 1,400 men and women who underwent coronary angiograms and were found to have at least one severely blocked coronary artery. After five years, those who were unmarried and who did not have at least one close confidante were over three times more likely to have died than people who were married, had one or more confidantes, or both.

The data on social networks and health is so compelling that Dean Ornish, M.D., who has published studies of his Lifestyle Program for Heart Disease (which includes elements of diet, exercise, meditation, and social support), recently wrote an entire book on the subject. In this well-documented work, *Love and Survival*, Ornish argues that love and intimacy are preeminent factors in health and well-being. "I am not aware of any other factor in medicine—not diet, not smoking, not stress, not genetics, not drugs, not surgery—that has a greater impact on our quality of life, incidence of illness, and premature death from all causes."

While parents, spouses, and children may represent the hub of our support systems, friends and siblings are the spokes that hold the wheel together. When we strengthen these spokes, we can keep traveling in good health and high spirits for a long and hardy lifetime.

WALK THE WALK, CUT THE TALK:
NURTURE THE BODY

There may be time when the people in your life (including friends and siblings) have you so stressed out, angry, or depressed that you need to redouble your commitment to a regular relaxation practice. Whether you choose meditation, body scan, progressive muscle relaxation, autogenic training, or any other method, regular practice may help you relate to your friend, brother, or sister with greater equanimity and compassion. It also helps to practice mini-relaxations when you're about to approach a friend for a tense conversation, or in the midst of a communication breakdown.

A fruitful way to nurture the body vis-à-vis friends and siblings is to join them in active forms of relaxation. Make time to go with your friend or sibling to a class in yoga, t'ai chi, or qi gong. Exercise classes can be energizing, revitalizing, and mood elevating; and taking them with friends and sisters offers a chance to do something healthy and fun together. One of my patients, Georgia, says, "When I exercise and go to yoga class with my friends, it recalls that childhood sense of play," she explained. "There you are, sweating together, throwing each other glances of encouragement, rolling your eyes as the instructor insists on a particularly demanding exercise or pose."

For Georgia, yoga with friends offers another satisfaction. "There's a sense of calm and serenity after yoga, and it's lovely to share that with someone you are close to. My friend and I leave the class in that same emotional space, which is a nice contrast to the typical feeling of being stressed or overburdened when you meet during a lunch break in a hectic coffee shop."

It may be counterintuitive, but in my experience the most powerful way to share relaxation with a friend or sibling is to take a mindful walk together. I say counterintuitive because mindful walks involve no speaking whatsoever, and talking is generally considered the hallmark of communication. Mindful walks reveal that there are other ways to communicate. You walk slowly, deliberately—mindfully—together, keeping your awareness anchored in the present while saying nothing. When possible, it's best to take mindful walks in peaceful natural environments, taking in the sights and sounds with all your senses.

Yes, women have the gift of empathy, and we support each other by talking out feelings and listening with a receptive ear. But women rarely offer each other the gift of silence; we're too busy talking. The long stretches of time spent together by couples allow for periods of silence—before bed, during meals, after making love. When women friends congregate there is often a sense of urgency—we want to share all the stories and iron out all the problems in one sitting. That's why mindful walks can be so comforting; the pressure to entertain or to hash it all out is absent, replaced by the sheer delight of sharing movement, and moments of sensory awareness, with someone you care about.

Truth or Dare: Nurture the Mind

Friends

When friendships are strained, we often revert to such automatic negative thoughts as, "She doesn't care about me." "She's driving me nuts with her problems." "She's a bitch." "She never listens to me."

Such thoughts often contain kernels of truth, but more often they are cognitive distortions. Friends can be disappointing, they sometimes don't listen, they certainly can drive us nuts. But in most intimate long-term friendships, we often waste time and energy with our negative or distorted thinking.

Consider the following sample restructurings; perhaps they apply to some of your friendships.

NEGATIVE THOUGHT: "She's a selfish bitch."

RESTRUCTURED THOUGHT: "I've been friends with her for years; why would I be friends with a 'selfish bitch' for so long? Actually, she's only like this occasionally. In fact, she has only been this angry and narcissistic since she's had so much trouble in her marriage and her job."

NEGATIVE THOUGHT: "She's driving me nuts with her problems."

RESTRUCTURED THOUGHT: "True, right now she is obsessed with her

problems with men and can't stop
talking about them. But she hasn't always
been this obsessed, and I have not really
let her know how unequal I think our
relationship has become. I guess she
must feel it's okay to drone on and on, so
I'm participating in the problem, as
well."

Follow these models to identify and transform your automatic negative thoughts regarding friendships. Of course, there are times when our negative thoughts represent parts of the truth. Friends who are enduringly self-centered, who never meet our needs, who cannot accept honest communication or tolerate differences, may not merit our trust. Once we apply cognitive restructuring to evaluate the veracity of our negative thoughts, we may need to reassess the friendship.

Ask yourself these questions:

1. Is the friendship nourishing, at least some of the time?
2. Is there a slight imbalance in the give-and-take equation, or is there a painful, complete disparity?
3. Has the deficit in this friendship always been present?

If the answers to these questions point to a problem in the relationship, then it is time to use assertiveness and communication skills to bring about change. If your efforts bear no fruit, it is probably time to move on.

Crises often bring out our friends' true colors. One of my patients, Margo, was in the midst of an ongoing medical crisis when she discovered that she could not count on one of her best friends, Allison. A week before the symptoms of an autoimmune disease became so debilitating that she landed in the hospital, Margo baby-sat for Allison's young daughter. That evening, Allison screamed at her over the phone about the Chinese food she'd served, which Allison's daughter didn't like. Margo reminded her friend that they'd had a previous phone conversation about what the daughter would eat, and Allison had said, "Absolutely anything." The sheer irrationality of Allison's phone attack was the final signal that Margo could not rely on Allison's judgment, let alone her support. This was the last straw in a relationship that had been deteriorating for years.

Letting go of unfulfilling or destructive friendships is itself a way to be self-nurturing. Some old friendships are worth holding on to for a lifetime; others become no more than a hook for feelings of nostalgia. It can be hard to let go of old friendships, but the fact that someone was your best friend at five does not necessarily mean you remain compatible at thirty-five. Cognitive restructuring—a systematized form of soul-searching—can help you figure out the basis of your friendships. The insights gained enable you to make decisions about which friendships to let go of and which to nurture with thoughtfulness and heartfulness.

Siblings

Cognitive restructuring of negative thoughts can also help regarding our sibling relationships. My relationship with my older sister Ricky, my only sibling, is a case in point.

When I entered graduate school for my doctorate in health psychology, one of the requirements was a stint in psychotherapy. I recall telling this to my family before returning to New York, and my sister followed me out to the car in something of a panic. "I'm really nervous about you going into therapy," she said. "You'll realize what a horrible older sister I was."

I was taken aback. "I don't perceive you as having been a horrible older sister," I replied. I did have memories of her teasing me. But I also remembered how much fun she was, and from my perspective, we supported each other most of the time. I explained this to Ricky as we stood outside in the driveway. For her, this became a memorable instance of cognitive restructuring. Clearly, she'd been saddled with guilt about the way she'd treated me. Once I shared my perception of her as a good older sister, and assured her that I'd let go of any resentment over her actions as a child, she began to release herself from the grip of guilt.

What about my own cognitive restructuring? It didn't seem necessary, because I wasn't harboring any bad feelings. But why not? When I delved deeper into my feelings about our relationship, I realized that over the years I'd been practicing cognitive restructuring all along.

I was a chubby child, which really bothered my father. He teased me about it quite a bit, and he encouraged my sister to tease me as well. Ricky, who is five years older, says she is haunted by these memories. But Ricky was very much my father's favorite, and she always sought his approval. Several years ago, while discussing these childhood episodes with Ricky, I had a flashback in which I saw my father clapping his hands and saying "Bravo!" as Ricky teased me. That memory, and my recognition that it was not an isolated event, helped me realize why I never blamed my sister for being mean to me. My father had set her up, and he'd set me up. My father thought that teasing me, and encouraging my sister to tease me, would help me lose weight. But what happened instead was that my father set us against each other. As a result of this insight, I never held my sister's actions against her.

My father was not at heart a cruel man, and I've since forgiven him for his insensitivity, which, I suspect, came from a lack of psychological awareness and, most likely, his own family experiences. But I always intuitively understood why Ricky harassed and sometimes hurt me. This allowed me to forgive her and to focus instead on her strengths, talents, and compassion. We also make each other laugh like no one else.

That key question of cognitive restructuring, "Where did this thought come from?," can lead to profound understanding. Here are several typical negative thoughts about siblings with sample restructurings. Use them to help you identify and transform your most powerful negative thoughts regarding your sibling relationships.

NEGATIVE THOUGHT: "My parents treated my brother better than me. I will always feel one-down in the eyes of my family—and myself."

RESTRUCTURED THOUGHT: "It's true that they treated my brother differently from me, but my reasoning about why—that he must be more talented and worthier—is wrong. He got more support for his intellectual and creative talents than I did, I now realize, because he was a boy. My parents bought into the misogynistic prejudices of their times; why should I continue to be plagued by their wrong-headed beliefs?"

NEGATIVE THOUGHT: "I know I treated my younger sister badly and she has not forgiven me. I let her down and she'll never let me get close to her again."

RESTRUCTURED THOUGHT: "Yes, I did abuse her but I now realize that I was taking out rage over abuse from our parents on my helpless younger sister. If I let her know that I understand what happened in our family, perhaps she'll come to forgive me and we can have the relationship I wish for. If she can't forgive me, at least I can forgive myself through an awareness of what happened to both of us when we were children, dependent upon our parents and subject to their hurtful behavior."

I include the brother example because many women feel inferior in their relationships with their brothers, often due to the disparity in treatment by parents, teachers, and peers. Restructurings like the above can gradually heal the hurts associated with unfair or unequal treatment.

I am often astonished by the potency of negative thoughts generated by sibling relationships. I think of Cary and Belinda, a couple who participated in one of my workshops for patients with infertility. Belinda, in her early forties, had an eight-year-old daughter and had been trying unsuccessfully for years to have a second child. The couple finally became pregnant, but she delivered the baby at twenty-four weeks and the baby died. Needless to say, it was an extraordinarily traumatic event for the couple. They joined our workshop a few months later, and during a cognitive restructuring exercise, Belinda shared this astonishing thought: "I have this weird thought that my baby died because I was a terrible older sister," she said.

Belinda believed she'd been unforgivably mean to her younger brother during childhood. Now, she felt, God's way of punishing her was to prevent her daughter from becoming an older sister to a new baby. This struck all of us in the group as a graphic example of an innocent person's needlessly blaming herself for a senseless tragedy.

I asked Belinda to put her negative thoughts to the cognitive test. Had she really been a terrible older sister? Yes, she remembers hitting and teasing and being mean to her baby brother. Had she ever asked her brother about this? Yes, several times, and her brother insisted that she'd been a great older sister. His strongest memories were of Belinda driving him everywhere as soon as she got her license, taking him to movies, ballgames, and her older friends' houses. Belinda's cognitive distortion was a magnification; she'd focused on a few incidents during an anguished phase in her childhood and turned them into a lifelong self-indictment.

We explored why Belinda would use this distorted thought to justify an even more devastating distortion—that God was punishing her by denying her daughter the joy of becoming an older sister. The group discussed how common it is for us to seek explanations—no matter how far-fetched—for inexplicable tragedies. Many of us would rather blame ourselves for a calamity than accept the hard reality that our loss occurred for no reason or purpose whatsoever.

Belinda's cognitive deciphering freed her from unnecessary self-blame over her baby's death. It also freed her from wrong assumptions about her treatment of her younger brother, which she experienced as a great weight being lifted from her soul. When it comes to our sibling relationships, cognitive restructuring can untangle the confusing complex of long-held misunderstandings and hurt feelings. So take the time to replace thoughts laden with self-blame, rage, and confusion. The result may be a longed-for transformation in our relations with our brothers and sisters.

BEYOND BITCH AND MOAN: NURTURE THE EMOTIONS

Sooner or later you've heard all your friends have to say. Then comes the tolerance of real love.

—Ned Rorem

Friends

Allow me to begin with a few generalizations about women that some may view as politically incorrect. With regard to friendships, women have certain strengths and certain weaknesses. Our strengths include empathy; the ability to articulate feelings; a facility for insight and intuition; the capacity to listen; the gift of gab. Our weaknesses include a tendency to wallow in suffering, shrink from confrontation, harbor jealousy, and engage in a subtle but sometimes destructive competitiveness.

I admit my generalizations border on stereotypes. I certainly know women who never whine and others who never empathize. But the old axiom that women are better at expressing emotion than men is largely true, even with the advent of the sensitive nineties man. We should celebrate this positive trait while recognizing its shadow side—what I call our "bitch and moan" tendency. Women seem vulnerable to ongoing negative self-thought and obsessive analysis of personal woundings (what author Caroline Myss calls "woundology"). While I would never cite this vulnerability to blame the female victims of trauma, many women fall prey to the "bitch and moan" pattern of rehashing negative events without meaningful catharsis, insight, or the prospect of real change. I've done it myself, and so have many patients and friends. Lots of men do it, too.

How can we stop wallowing? The answer begins with cognitive restructuring. We're better off when we grapple with the underlying causes of our suffering and work toward solutions, when our friends are active listeners and advisers rather than passive sounding boards for a stream of complaints. When we move deeply into emotion, we certainly need friends who remain quiet and listen with compassion. But we also need friends willing to challenge our assumptions—to encourage our new realizations and behavioral shifts so we don't get stuck in our own personal Groundhog's Day (remember the Bill Murray film in which he relives the same dreary events over and over?).

So how do we deal with friends who bitch and moan? Sometimes we collude with them by shrinking from honest confrontation. We fear being perceived as intolerant or impatient—a "bad friend" who's not a good listener. Yes, we don't want to hurt their feelings, but, more to the point, we don't want to be spurned by a wounded friend. It helps to remember that we can "confront" with kindness and empathy. When we follow the basic communication skills of assertiveness (rather than passivity, aggression, or passive aggression), we get our point across without causing gratuitous pain. And sometimes, a carefully timed and articulated piece of hard-nosed advice can draw us closer to a friend whose complaining is really a call for serious help.

This was Francesca's strategy, one of my stressed-out patients who'd become fed up with her friend Susan's relentless husband-bashing. According to Susan, her spouse, Harold, was forgetful, controlling, and utterly preoccupied with his work. But ·Susan was consumed by her discontent with Harold and hardly ever talked about anything else. Francesca longed for the earlier days of her friendship with Susan, when they enjoyed social occasions, laughed through countless lunches, and practiced aerobics in lockstep at a local health club.

Francesca tried cognitive restructuring. If Harold was so terrible, why had Susan married him? Her answer: He *used to be* intelligent, witty, and ambitious, but he was fast losing those qualities. Francesca recognized the tactic: Susan exaggerated every incident in order to sustain her case against her husband. Had his wit and intelligence really disappeared? Francesca wondered whether it was really all Harold's fault: Had Susan's anger also poisoned the marriage? Francesca knew Harold well, and while she saw truth in her friend's complaints, she thought the couple had been good for each other in the past, and might be again. Susan's repetitive, self-righteous fury, she thought, was blocking any chance of progress in the marriage, not to mention their friendship.

With few options left, Francesca ceased playing the dreary role of sounding board, and shifted to active participant in the drama. She finally said to Susan, "It hurts me to listen to you bash Harold. First, it's difficult to hear you spin your wheels, especially when you're in such pain. But it's also painful to me, since I feel we're losing other dimensions of our friendship. You can take my advice—you and Harold love each other and could resolve these tensions if you get professional help. Or don't take my advice; that's fine, too. But we should put a cap on the time we spend talking about Harold. One third of every visit, and that's it. Then let's talk about other issues, my problems, and do some fun stuff together."

Susan later admitted that she'd been so used to Francesca as the sympathetic ear that she was startled by the sudden appearance of Francesca the aggrieved friend. At first, Susan experienced her comments as wounding. But Susan did not want to lose the friendship, and she did her best to curtail her repetitive complaints about Harold. A year later, Francesca told me that Susan and Harold had entered couples counseling and were working hard to iron out their conflicts. The two friends were spending even more time together, and the intimacy and high spirits of their earlier friendship had been reclaimed.

Think of your wallowing friend (or yourself, as the case may be) as a long-playing record. Under normal circumstances, you're able to listen to the music without interruption. But when the record skips, and all you hear is that repeating loop of screechy sound, you need to take action—advancing the tone arm past the scratch so you can once again hear the music. An honest reflection to a suffering friend can get her over the hump that keeps her stuck.

Taking such risks are acts of autonomy, authenticity, and care for one's friend. As Christine Downing once wrote, "There is space within sisterhood for likeness and difference, for the subtle differences that challenge and delight; there is space for disappointment—and surprise."

It can also be emotionally healing to write about a troubled friendship. You may simply wish to write out your thoughts and feelings about the friendship, or about recent events that were hurtful or bewildering. I often suggest that women write letters to friends, particularly when the friendship is a prolonged source of suffering. You can send the letter or not. If you do, it may be an opportunity to share concerns and feelings, including anger, that seem too threatening in a one-on-one encounter. Often, however, such letters are forms of blood-letting that may be valuable only to you as a form of release. Ask yourself whether the letter you've written serves the larger purpose of better relations before you decide to send it.

One of my infertility patients was having a terrible time with her friend who was a single mother. This woman did not seem to comprehend the turbulence and sorrow the infertile friend experienced on a daily basis. I suggested that they consider writing each other letters in which they fully expressed their thoughts and feelings. This practice enables each of them to work through their emotions and to digest the whole of the other's experience, not just one "sound bite" at a time. In this instance, the process worked beautifully. My patient wrote about the pain she'd endured: "I feel like my life has been on hold for five years. I live in cycles of despair, and I can hardly see light at the end of the tunnel." Her friend wrote back about how difficult it was to be a single mother: "Some days I just want to escape from it all." My patient came to understand how her friend's immense problems as a mother had blinded her to the anguish of infertility, while her friend finally saw the truth of my patient's struggle and the anguish infertility had caused. Reading the letters reunited the long-term friends who had only wished, all along, to bridge the growing divide before it became a permanent gulf.

Siblings

Marnie's siblings created a family within the family—a cocoon of love and support in an environment of fear and hostility. Her old-world parents were tyrannical, and Marnie, who describes her mother as "crazy," was physically and emotionally abused on a regular basis. In later life, Marnie was not only disinherited, she was subject to regular fits of verbal humiliation by her mother. Her younger brother William had multiple birth defects and was not tyrannized in the same way. Marnie's older sister Lisa avoided the worst punishments by maintaining a façade of sweetness and serenity. While Marnie took the brunt of the abuse, family life was a nightmare for all three siblings.

In this fearful atmosphere, the three drew together and supported each other from early childhood into adulthood. William was the one sibling who was not a target of physical abuse, but he empathized with his sisters, and he did everything he could to stop the parents from meting out harsh punishments. Marnie looked to William as "her protector" when she was young, and today she looks to William as an inspiring role model. He's succeeded in business and he maintains a buoyant spirit in the face of severe physical handicaps that have only worsened with time. Marnie also admires and turns to her sister Lisa, who has gradually grown from a passive supplicant to an assertive defender of herself and her siblings. All of them treat each other with a tenderness and concern forged in the heartless and hostile environment of their parents' home.

Of course, every family is different. Connecting with our siblings requires us to consider our unique familial circumstances. How siblings relate over the course of decades is determined by a mix of factors: assigned family roles, personality differences, birth order, parental expectations, and peer group pressures. While there are no simple rules on how best to nurture the emotional side of our sibling relationships, I have found certain guidelines to be helpful.

First, it's critical to acknowledge both our similarities and differences with our siblings. Problems arise when we expect a sibling to react and behave the way we do, which is usually based on the mistaken assumption that since we come from the same family, our values and way of thinking will be the same. Conversely, problems also arise when we *underestimate* our shared values and experiences, when we forget how much we do, in fact, have in common.

When we feel distant or alienated from a sibling, or continually angry over perceived insults or misunderstandings, it helps to ask ourselves this key question: What are my expectations of our relationship now? Often, siblings who are close as children assume they will be lifelong friends, but when marriages and jobs take them in different directions, both geographically and creatively, the previously tight bonds can loosen. The resulting disappointment or even anger can cause relationships to fray, at which point it's important to establish new expectations from our siblings. I see this all the time with patients: over the course of decades, we often take wildly divergent paths from our brothers and sisters. In these instances, it's an illusion to think we can hold onto the old kind of closeness.

If we're willing to restructure our expectations, we can have a new sort of closeness, one that retains the best aspects of what we shared in childhood while respecting the fact that our directions have diverged and our needs have changed. I've experienced this with my sister, Ricky. As the older sister, she was always my teacher. (In fact, she later became a math teacher.) For decades, I looked to her for advice and support and she willingly and generously offered it. In more recent years, Ricky has had cause to seek my counsel as a health professional working in a hospital, plying me for medical information and contacts. Indeed, in the past decade she's come to me for advice more often than I've gone to her. At the same time, in moments of emotional turmoil I have turned to her, and then it feels like we're back to our family pattern. It is the flexibility in our relationship that has kept us close throughout the years.

———————

When you experience a disturbing rift with a sibling, all too frequently the cause is a profound misunderstanding of the other's experience within the family. One patient, Hannah, had trouble with her older brother, Sam, who had been adopted four years before she was born. Sam felt that Hannah was favored by their parents because she was the biological child they had desired for so many years. Hannah understood Sam's feelings, since she thought they were rooted in truth—in many respects their parents *had* favored her. (To Sam's dismay, Hannah was dubbed the "miracle child." Hannah didn't much like this designation, either.) But she also thought that Sam overlooked the pain and pressure associated with being the favorite—the high expectations she could never meet. As adults, they talked about their different roles within the family, and in so doing they gained deeper understanding of each other's struggles, and a more mature closeness. Hannah acknowledged that Sam had suffered a form of emotional neglect, and Sam recognized that Hannah had suffered in her lifelong effort to fulfill her parents' image of her as the brilliant star in the family.

When you have trouble with a sibling, consider sitting down with him or her and asking this question: What was your experience in the family? Too often, we assume we understand our sibling's experience without having even one probing conversation. Take the time to share your memories and experiences, and give your brother or sister the same opportunity.

As with friends, you can also use letter writing to explore and express emotions about your sibling relationships. I see this all the time in Ann Landers: "I haven't spoken to my brother in ten years. What can I do?" Well, write him a letter and get to the crux of what you believe is the problem, the issue or event in the past that has precipitated the separation. If you have a problem with a sibling, whether you're estranged or remain relatively close, you may wish to write two versions: the letter you *don't* send and one you do. Start with the one you don't send, using it as a means to explore unreleased emotions—every shade of sorrow, rage, confusion, resentment. For the one you send, be honest but not self-indulgent; articulate your positions and feelings without finger-pointing.

Here are guidelines (Exercise 1) for the letter you don't send, based on psychologist James Pennebaker's model for healing confessions.

Then I suggest you try writing a letter from your sibling's point of view (Exercise 2). Finally, I suggest guidelines for writing a second version of the letter from your own point of view, one you may be able to send (Exercise 3).

1. Write your deepest thoughts and feelings about your sibling and relationship with him or her. If tied to a particular event in the past, write about what happened and your feelings at the time. What do you want to say to your brother or sister about your past and present relationship?

2. Repeat the first writing exercise, but this time put yourself in the shoes of your sibling. Write what you imagine are his feelings, perceptions, experiences, and perspectives about your relationship.

3. Write out your thoughts and feelings to your sibling but take care to consider her feelings. Use "I" statements that communicate feelings and take responsibility for your point of view, rather than "you" statements (i.e., you did this to me, you are a selfish jerk, etc.) that foist blame and place yourself in the position of victim.

Share your view of your family history and how you feel it affected your relationship. Write about how you've changed; how you'd do things differently today; your hopes for your future relationship.

A SECOND FAMILY:
NURTURE THE SELF/SPIRIT

Marnie, my patient who forged close ties with her brother and sister to sustain herself through a hellish childhood, also wove together a web of supportive friendships that nourished her throughout her late adolescence and adulthood. Here are her reflections on friendships in her college years:

> The message I got from my parents was, "You're not okay," and my college friends wrapped their arms around me and loved me and told me I was wonderful and nurtured me and made me feel okay. That's still true of my college roommate. We were together at a

benefit recently, and she said to me, "I don't want you to go near that mother." Her understanding goes back nineteen years. She remembers me sitting on my bed crying when everyone's parents came up for parents' weekend, except mine. When I would walk into the Dean of Students Office, where students would always congregate, I was everyone's mother hen. I solved everyone's problems, overfunctioning on every level. I once had this very astute psychologist tell me to sit down for one minute. He said, "What goes on behind that smile? What are you about?" And I burst into tears. This person had stopped me and said, "Life just can't be that perfect." So I regurgitated my whole life story. He responded, "Why aren't you a drug addict or prostitute?" I said, "Because of my sister and brother and friends." That's what has kept me from going the other way. And it's still true twenty-five years later.

Marnie's story underscores how we can nurture self and spirit through friendship. She'd formed a second family that, in her case, eclipsed her parents in meeting her needs. I have many patients and acquaintances who've created second families comprised of friends and neighbors when their families of origin are dysfunctional, disappointing, or both. These second families are authentically nurturing support networks forged out of love and choice. "God gave us our relatives," said Ethel Watts Mumford. "Thank God we can choose our friends."

Neglecting friendship carries a price we may not acutely feel from one year to the next, but it's a hefty price nonetheless. A common form of neglect occurs whenever we form a new romantic partnership or get married. I've seen it happen with patients, friends, and relatives: a woman falls head over heels for a man and virtually dumps her female friends. Once the relationship stabilizes, she wakes up to the realization that he can't meet all her needs. She's suddenly hit with a second realization: Her friends are no longer there for her. Frequently, her own withdrawal was the real cause of their actual or emotional absence. Unless we reestablish the balance between our romantic relationship and our friendships, the latter may wither on the vine.

In practical terms, when we become deeply involved in a romantic relationship, we can prevent the dissolution of friendships by letting our friends know that although our bar-hopping days may be over, it is still important to spend time together.

We must hold fast to the recognition that a significant other will never fulfill all the needs of our multifaceted selves; we need a variety of friends to do that. Three or four may do; it's not necessary to be queen of the social whirl. But we'll lose our web of supportive friendships if we don't nurture them with loving kindness. To nurture our social networks, we must remain available to our friends, and we must let them know when we need them. To borrow a wise saying from mind-body pioneer George Solomon, M.D., "If you don't communicate with your support system, then the system isn't supportive."

Among the most powerful ways to nurture self and spirit vis-à-vis friendships is to join groups with other women. In days of old, women friends and neighbors sat around stitching quilts and sweaters and baby blankets as they chatted about their families and dreams. Or they joined coffee klatches where gossip and gab were raised to the level of high art. It's a sad irony of modern life that most women never join groups until they've been diagnosed with something serious, like breast cancer or substance abuse. Why should we have to get breast cancer to fulfill our need for sisterhood?

I recently joined a Friday afternoon play group with my young daughter, Sarah. It gives her an opportunity to play with peers, and it gives me a chance to talk with other mothers. Most of my friends work full-time and have children older than Sarah. I thoroughly enjoy sitting in the park, watching our kids while talking to this group of women, all of whom are smart and funny and willing to share their experiences as mothers with young children. I imagine it's as close as I'll get to the sense of community my mother and grandmother had when they were young.

Be creative in your decisions about self-nurturing pursuits with friends. Have a "chick's night out"—get dressed up and go to a restaurant with three or four friends, then see a movie your male friends or mates might never select. Go mountain hiking, cross-country skiing, or rowboating. It's always great to sweat with friends, whether at a gym or a dance or aerobics class. Make a trip with one or more friends to the latest art exhibit, dance, or musical concert. (One of my friends bought a ballet subscription for two every season, and took a different friend to each program.) Sign up for a class on how to cook ethnic food or bake French pastries. Take an interior decorating or photography class. Convince a friend to join you in learning how to play a musical instrument, no matter how offbeat—drums, banjo, or electric guitar, if one of them strikes your fancy.

If time is an issue for you, try the following:

- Make a point of telephoning at least one friend once a week.
- As often as you can, socialize with friends whose children are the same age as yours so that you have a chance to talk while your kids play together.
- Take advantage of a free hour to go out with a friend for an ice cream cone, frozen yogurt, or a quick cup of coffee.

You can also organize self-nurturing activities for larger gatherings than two or three. We vastly underestimate the healing power of groups and the immeasurable value of feeling that we're part of a community of women. I am heartened by the new kinds of groups cropping up to meet these needs—the reading clubs, art appreciation gatherings, and creativity circles. A prime example is Julia Cameron's book *The Artist's Way*, which has spurred the formation of "Artist's Way" groups—small cohorts of women coming together to discuss and practice ways to realize their creativity.

I recommend "self-nurture" groups, in which women friends join together to talk about how they can become more self-nurturing, and practice the hands-on exercises in self-nurturance that I have developed. With this book in hand, you can start such a group, focusing on one chapter each time you meet. Consider these suggestions for how you might conduct such a group:

Start the group with a relaxation exercise, such as the body scan, perhaps playing an audiotape for guidance. Then you might discuss how you put the self-nurture suggestions into practice, where you feel you've succeeded and where you feel you need more focus and support. Take fifteen minutes to do a writing exercise from that chapter (theme) and discuss the thoughts and feelings that surfaced. You might conclude by sharing specific commitments to self-nurture you hope to honor in the coming weeks. Let loose your sense of play; enjoy the time with friends and allow your collective imaginations to seize on new ways to nurture yourselves in solitude and relationship.

You can also turn your self-nurture meetings into field trips. Summer is a good time for country walks, excursions to a lake or beach, gatherings in a nearby park, or, if your group is small enough, long drives to places in the country you've always wanted to explore. In the fall, go apple picking or take yourselves out to an ice cream parlor and indulge yourselves. Could there be any more appropriate bunch of people with whom to do nurturing things than your self-nurture group?

Siblings

While my sister Ricky and I are very close, our hectic nineties lives and families seem to conspire to prevent us from spending time alone together. Though I can drive to her house in forty-five minutes, arranging a one-on-one visit often seems as unlikely as copping a ticket to a Boston Celtics game. It's neither her fault nor mine, though perhaps we could make an even more concerted effort than we do. We talk on the phone regularly, sometimes pouring out our hearts over recent troubles or disappointments. We get together for most major holidays. But I still would like more time alone with Ricky, because she knows me better than anyone else. We share sensibilities and belly laughs so intense we've been known to fall off furniture.

I've observed that, for most of us, as we get older and move in different directions, it takes a special effort for us to overcome our hectic lives and schedules to fit in time with our brothers and sisters. But if something besides your busy life keeps getting in the way, have an exploratory talk with your sibling. Are there family secrets or painful memories you think you can avoid by keeping your distance? Do you harbor unacknowledged anger or guilt about your sibling, and fear a confrontation? Do you feel he's disappointed you, or you him? Do your best to find out what's getting in the way. You don't want to wake up in thirty years and realize you've lost a sibling due to your own evasiveness or timidity.

Find fun things to do together. You might want to engage in some of the activities you enjoyed as children, as long as they don't require you to regress completely to a five-year-old state. For example,

- Go roller blading, winter sledding, or skiing.
- Play backyard badminton, volleyball, or shoot hoops.
- Play card games that breed conversation—Gin Rummy, Bridge, or Hearts.

- Drag out old board games stashed away in your family's attic—Monopoly, Risk, Life, or Parcheesi—and reminisce while you play.
- If both you and a sibling are married, go out as a foursome. Try a dinner out or even a vacation together to get to know your brother- or sister-in-law better. Too often, you only see siblings and their mates in the chaotic context of larger family dinners and holiday gatherings.

No matter what the activity, try to find your way back to the playfulness and humor you've shared with your sibling in the past. Probably no one else can make you laugh like a brother or sister—and that's something to be cherished.

Reminiscing is among the greatest pleasures of siblings. My sister and I traveled a great deal as children since my father's academic positions took him all over the world. We spent many summers in foreign locales, ranging from Israel to South America. But the best memories Ricky and I have were vacations spent with our cousins, the Rosenthals. Time with the Rosenthals meant constant laughter, and all these years later, Ricky and I still enjoy recalling our shared experiences.

One of our favorite family stories occurred during the summer when I was fifteen and she was twenty. My parents had rented a cottage on a small island off the coast of Massachusetts for a two-week vacation. They slept in the bedroom while my sister and I slept on a pullout couch in the living room. We had to put out the garbage by nine o'clock in the morning on Mondays and Thursdays, since the garbage truck arrived precisely on time. One Thursday morning, my parents had overslept and my sister and I heard the loud sputter of the garbage truck coming down the street. The sound must have awakened them, since my father ran full-speed out of the bedroom in his canary-yellow pajamas. He grabbed several garbage bags and ran outside at top speed to greet the garbage truck—just in time. My sister and mother and I burst into laughter at the sight of my father, always the formal university professor, dashing about in his yellow pajamas in the bright morning sunshine. A few weeks later my father had to buy new pajamas; he could no longer don the canary-yellow ones without our breaking up. It was a story my sister and I told at his funeral, and even then we could not stop ourselves from giggling at the memory of him that morning a quarter-century ago.

The memories we share with our siblings are the very stuff of our mutual identities. Reliving them can remind us of who we are, as individuals and as members of the family nexus. We can also enjoy the company of our brothers and sisters at church, synagogue, or mosque. As we age, and grandparents, aunts, uncles, and parents pass away, we may feel a greater need to worship together. The religious rituals of childhood can be renewed or replaced with ones that hold more meaning for us as adults who can finally make our own choices about spiritual practice. The pursuit of prayer and spiritual awakening can sometimes be a powerful way to reclaim intimacy with the people who may know us better than anyone else on the planet.

Fall

Auspicious Beginnings

8

JOY AT WORK:

SAFEGUARDING SOUL

ON THE JOB

☙ ❧

We must pay more attention to the kind and quality of work at which we spend our days, our weeks, our lives. It's not just about jobs, or even well-paying jobs. It's about meaningful work. We need work that is good for body, mind, and spirit; work that sustains family and community; work that connects us with and helps us protect the natural world.

—Andrew Kimbrell

AS A LAWYER specializing in mental health, Marion defends many people—usually mothers whose children have been legally removed from the home. Every day, she fights fierce battles on their behalf in phone conversations, conferences, and courtrooms. "There is so much emotion in the office," says Marion. "These cases have become very difficult for me." A perfect example is the thirty-seven-year-old mother whose substance abuse led a judge to rescind her parental custody rights. As Marion prepared her appeal, the mother broke down: "I'm trying so hard to stay sober. The only reason I keep going is because I love these kids so much." Marion ached for the woman, whose heartbreak was as undeniable as her addiction. She ached, too, for the father of a nine-year-old boy who landed in jail on tax evasion and lost custody of his son. Marion had to tell the man he had virtually no chance of winning on appeal, which meant he wouldn't be permitted to see the boy until he was eighteen. Marion's caseload is overflowing with such emotionally charged stories.

For a long time, Marion's way of coping with her workaday stress made matters worse. "I would dissociate from my body," she said. "If I felt hunger, I ignored it. If my shoulders were tense—it all goes to my shoulders—I wouldn't know it until I got home. In order to function at work, I ignored my emotional temperature. I would just keep on whipping myself into a frenzy."

I encouraged Marion to start taking her "temperature," her emotional, physical, and spiritual state of being at work and at home. "I took a step back and realized how emotionally loaded my profession is. I started asking myself, 'What's making me feel this way?' and 'Is there a better way to handle the difficult feelings that come up?' "

Marion confronted the fact that her work experiences were powerfully reminiscent of her own emotional history. As I discussed in Chapter 3, her mother had been repeatedly institutionalized, and Marion ran away from home at thirteen, right after the sudden death of her father, "the only solid person in my life." She recalls the guardianship hearing in which her mother was deemed unfit, and Marion was remanded to the custody of her foster parents. "I witnessed the court officers taking my mother away in restraints," she says. "I'd been forced by the judge to say in open court, 'I can't live with my mom anymore.' " Marion still has a troubled relationship with her mother, though years of psychotherapy have helped.

But in her professional life, Marion struggled to patch up families as ravaged as her own, which was undeniably draining. I encouraged her to pay closer attention to the effects of her work on her emotions and spirit. She began to recognize when a client's circumstance tripped a wire in her psyche, and instead of dissociating by working more frantically, Marion took a break, a deep breath, and acknowledged her feelings at that moment. "I've become more tuned in to my emotions," says Marion. "When I have an anguished conversation with a client, I know I need to go outside for a walk, or talk it through with one of my partners. I draw clearer boundaries with my clients, and I keep checking in with myself."

Marion uses her body as a guide; when she becomes frantic or disconnected, she knows it's time to do something to nurture herself. "I can't completely control the outcome of my cases," she says. "But I do have some control over my state of mind. When I get home, I meditate, get into a bathtub, light a candle, and focus on my breathing. I think about how blessed I am. My husband is in the next room watching the *Lehrer News Hour*; we don't have money worries; he loves me, and I love him. In that moment, there isn't a single thing wrong with my life."

Whether your job is emotionally overwhelming, physically demanding, intellectually challenging, or just plain difficult, self-nurture can safeguard body and soul. As in Marion's case, you can take your emotional and physical temperature on the job, then develop strategies for self-care that meet your needs.

In this era of multiple roles for women, which can also include multiple jobs, work-related stress is at an all-time high. And the jobs themselves are more pressure-packed. In a recent poll, 88 percent of workers said their jobs require them to work longer (up from 70 percent two decades ago), and 68 percent complained of having to work at greater speeds (up from 50 percent in 1977). You can rely on relaxation techniques, both at home and in the workplace, to release yourself from the grip of work-related stressors. You can supplant self-doubting, self-defeating thought patterns that hold you back from realizing success in your career. You can work through emotional blocks to discovering your creative potential and self-esteem at work, and develop strong communication skills with coworkers and employers that will see you through the inevitable tensions that arise. Finally, you can discover or rediscover meaning in your work, whether by changing your psychospiritual outlook regarding your current job, or by changing jobs altogether. Read on.

GIVE ME A BREAK!
RELAXATION AT WORK

Every Wednesday, I participate in work-related meetings at the Beth Israel Deaconess Medical Center. This includes an hour-long executive committee meeting followed by an hour-long staff meeting. Frequently, the issues presented at the first meeting are repeated at the second meeting. While this is nobody's fault, it frustrates me nevertheless. I am an extremely concrete person, and for better or worse, I lose patience during prolonged analyses of problems that call out for some practical solution. Sometimes I can move the dialogue forward, but often I can't. While I don't hold these discussions against my esteemed colleagues, I still experience a mixture of boredom and frustration that sets off my fight-or-flight response—leaving me tense and restless.

In such stressful circumstances, I could easily make two gargantuan mistakes. One would be to try to control the meetings myself (or try to sneak out!). The other would be to believe that I should change my personality. Once I accept that I can do neither, I'm left with a simpler solution. I can change my own inner response during the meetings. How so? The easiest way for me is to practice mini-relaxations.

Practice Minis

The wonder of minis, and the reason they are so useful at work, is that they are stress-busting techniques you can practice without having to sit quietly in an enclosed space with your eyes closed. You can practice minis in a meeting, at your desk, even in the middle of a stressful chat with your boss. You stop, breathe deeply into your abdomen, making certain that your diaphragm moves down, causing expansion of your belly. In your mind, you can perform one of the simple counting exercises that help prolong inhalation and exhalation (see pages 43–44). If the counting distracts you, it isn't absolutely necessary. You just need to shift from shallow chest breathing to deep diaphragmatic breathing.

Minis remind me that I can control my own stress response. I don't have to remain helpless against my own adrenaline rush when I get antsy. My shift to abdominal breathing calms me down and puts my focus where it belongs—on my own well-being. I find minis even more useful when my day goes completely awry, a less common event but one that is obviously more stressful than the usual Wednesday meetings.

I often give talks at conferences about my research into mind-body techniques for women's health conditions, such as PMS, menopausal symptoms, and infertility. Every so often, an audience member asks a question that is not just critical but outright hostile. I find these moments difficult; my heart rate increases and I can feel my face flush. My husband suggested that I pause and take a long, slow, deep breath—a mini-mini—before answering the question. It gives me a moment to break the stress response, clear my mind, and offer the least reactive and most thoughtful reply.

Use minis whenever a boss or coworker provokes you with irritating or hostile comments. If you think you're being harassed or abused, take considered, assertive action. But if you're dealing with the personality quirks of people you must deal with on a daily basis, focus on your own internal responses, using relaxation techniques to retain your equilibrium and protect yourself from the ravages of your own stress response.

Throughout your workday, continually check in with yourself regarding your stress level and its effect on your breathing. Relatively shallow breathing is one of the best barometers of stress, anxiety, boredom, and exhaustion. If you're anxious and have reverted to shallow breathing, mini-relaxations nip the stress response in the bud. They bring a fresh, cleansing breath deep into the lungs, short-circuiting the vicious cycle of internal stress and impoverished breathing. The first time you practice a mini on the job—in the presence of coworkers or higher-ups—you'll be delighted to discover how much control you can exercise over your own psychophysical well-being in the midst of your workday activities.

Ease the Aching Body-Mind (Body Scan and PMR)

It's four o'clock and you've reached the nadir of your day, that time when mental overload is accompanied by fatigue, aches, pains, and general malaise. You've been stuck in one sitting position for too long, concentrating too hard, forgetting your body's needs for refreshment, relaxation, movement, fresh air, and water. All you know is your symptoms. You reach for an aspirin, close your eyes, head for the water cooler, take a three-minute nap . . . but nothing you do relieves the strain or the symptoms.

I hear this scenario constantly. My stressed-out patients contend with severe headaches, backaches, shoulder aches, tendinitis, bursitis, wrist pain, sciatica, pins and needles, and flare-ups of arthritis. Less concretely, they suffer from chronic exhaustion, dizziness, low energy, and difficulty concentrating. Typically, these symptoms can be caused by continually tight muscles, which result from poor posture, shallow breathing, and the persistent fight-or-flight response associated with work pressures and interpersonal conflicts on the job. Whether you work in an office, restaurant, retail store, or construction site, your job can present emotional or physical challenges and constraints that leave an imprint on your body.

You can't cure all these problems at once. But you can practice forms of relaxation that release muscular tensions, which may offer quick relief from a wide range of physical symptoms. The body scan and progressive muscle relaxation (PMR) are gentle ways to nurture the beleaguered body/mind when the burdens of work take their toll.

You can't readily practice body scan or PMR in the middle of a meeting. All you need, however, is to find ten to fifteen minutes during your day when you can close the door to your office or take an outdoor break. Sit quietly and scan the body from head to toe, focusing on areas of tension during the in-breath, releasing tension on the out-breath. The "scan" procedure grounds you back into the body, alerting you to areas of contraction that you can relax with a sweeping, gentle awareness. As Steven Levine points out, when we sweep the body with awareness we bring kindness, mercy, and relaxation to muscles tightened by awkward postures, overwork, job-related pressures, and frozen emotional states.

PMR adds a concrete element to the body scan that is immensely helpful for people plagued by deep muscular tensions. If you suffer from intense or constant headaches, backaches, and shoulder aches, PMR can help you to identify and loosen the taut muscular bundles that cause you pain. During PMR, deliberately tighten each area of the body; when you purposely release tension from those areas, the feeling of relief is often more noticeable—and striking. PMR helps blood flow and respiration while reducing the effects of stress by eliciting the relaxation response. Many patients report a dramatic reduction of the frequency and intensity of their headaches, backaches, and other musculoskeletal symptoms. All of which helps to restore their capacity for playfulness, creativity, and joy on the job.

Combine Relaxation with Pleasure and Contact

It's the kiss of death to sit at a desk for eight or ten hours without moving, breathing fresh air, or giving your mind a rest from its narrowly trained focus on work matters. Get out and take a mindful walk!

I tell this to my hard-working patients and friends, and I almost always hear the same complaint: "But I just don't have time." This all-purpose excuse is sometimes also true. But instead of living out this assumption at work, where we never have enough time for *anything,* we can help ourselves through creative piggy-backing. One of my patients, Renata, was feeling draggy and disconnected at her job as an administrator at an HMO. She found a perfect solution. On good weather days, she spent half of her lunch break eating and the other half with a coworker roller blading in a nearby park. For Renata, roller blading carried multiple benefits: pleasure, exercise, relaxation, time with friends.

After hours of paperwork, roller blading reminded her that she had a body. And she made a point of skating mindfully, appreciating the moment-to-moment sensations: the wind at her face, her calf muscles flexing, the fleeting visual impressions of hanging trees, green landscapes, and people gliding by. It was also a chance to do something fun with her friend. Renata always felt refreshed and renewed by the time she returned to her office. Not all of us have parks—or the leg muscles—for roller blading, but we should be able to find a venue for modest exercise and time outdoors with friends.

In the spirit of self-nurture, there is time for companionship and time for solitude, as well. A few years ago, I was coping with several life challenges during a particularly harsh winter. There is a river behind the hospital where I work, and every day I took a mindful stroll outdoors, feeding the flock of ducks that gather by the river bank. Though it was cold, I needed the fresh air and the time alone to gather my thoughts and restore my spirit.

Create Your Own Relaxation Rituals

Eileen is a high-powered money manager, working sixty hours a week trading stocks for her clients. That doesn't count the twenty additional hours she devotes to nonprofit work. When she first came to me, Eileen complained not only of burnout, but an alarming set of symptoms. Her speech would inexplicably fail her, causing odd slips of the tongue, as when she was talking to a client and said "bond" when she meant to say "stock." She either couldn't find the right word, or the wrong word came tumbling out. Her memory was also a problem. "One time, a client told me to buy a thousand shares of a particular stock," Eileen recalled. "Weeks later I checked his account and I noticed that I'd never bought the thousand shares. I had to figure out the price he would have gotten when he made the request, and make good on the difference." This had not been an isolated incident.

Eileen had wisely gone for medical tests—MRIs, CAT scans, complete neurologic workups. The neurologists frightened her with talk of "demyelinating nerve cells," and a variety of disturbing diagnoses. "They tried to tell me I had everything from aphasia to multiple sclerosis to epilepsy."

Although I could add nothing to the medical speculation, when

Eileen described her work overload, I suggested that her daily pressures might be exacerbating her symptoms. This theory hit home when we figured out that her slips of the tongue and lapses of memory only happened on the job! They were not occurring with her husband or friends outside the office. Eileen grasped the intensity of her work stress once she tuned into her body-mind through relaxation. "I realized that I hold my breath all day," she says. "I was barely inhaling or exhaling. Not only that, I have chips in my teeth from constant grinding."

Eileen combined several relaxation techniques into a custom-tailored mind-body program. She brings body scan and imagery tapes with her to work, and when the going gets tough she locks herself in an empty room and drops into deep relaxation. "One minute I'm trading stocks furiously, the next minute I'm sitting by the ocean." Eileen relies on an audiotape of ocean imagery, as well as a tape of classical music overlaid with ocean sounds. She also uses a guided body-scan tape, and she practices minis all day long. Eileen elicits the relaxation response before, during, and after her work day.

Within a few weeks, Eileen's slips of the tongue and mind had improved. Her memory and articulation became sharper. The clear correlation between her relaxation practice and her symptomatic improvement motivates Eileen to keep using the body scan, minis, and ocean imagery every day of her life. (She still consults her doctors on a regular basis, although right now she requires no treatment.) Eileen is amazed by the sheer power of stress to exacerbate a neurologic dysfunction, and equally amazed by the power of relaxation to promote healing.

COMMITMENT, CONTROL, AND CHALLENGE: NURTURE THE MIND AT WORK

For some women, negative thoughts about work, whether they center on the daily grind or the big picture of career aspirations, are the most intolerable, inescapable inner voices they must battle. Consider this sample list of common, automatic negative thoughts about work and career:

I can't do this job.
I'm not smart enough.
The men in this company get the raises and promotions.

My weight problem holds me back on the job.

My creativity at work is blocked.

My coworkers are jealous of me, and they talk behind my back.

My boss doesn't appreciate my talents and skills.

I screwed up on my last assignment, so I'll never get another opportunity.

My colleague is much more skilled; I'll never live up to her standards.

If I don't ace this project, my boss will lose all respect for me.

I know for certain that I am getting fired.

I'll never have a job that pays me enough money to have what I want in life.

I'll never have a career that gives me meaning and joy.

Which of these thoughts eat away at you? Write them down, or any other negative thoughts that hound you. When you separate the truths from the self-criticisms, you can overcome the blocks to self-esteem, creative expression, and spiritual connectedness on the job.

Veronica was new in her high-pressure job as an associate editor at a women's magazine. Her boss was a rather distant man, a poor communicator with a short temper. In my cognitive work with Veronica, she uncovered a cluster of pernicious negative thoughts that had plagued her during her six months on the job: "I can't do this work," "I'm late with projects because I keep screwing up," "My boss has a low opinion of me."

We looked inside this cluster, and found a nasty core of illogical and unrealistic assumptions. Veronica's boss was tough, and he had expected too much of her in a short time. He judged her harshly, but not as harshly as Veronica feared. When she spoke to coworkers, she realized that he treated most employees the same way. She also recognized, with much compassion for herself, that she was especially vulnerable to angry authoritarian men. "No wonder this man scares you!" I remarked. Veronica had been late with projects, not because she was "screwing up," but because she was a perfectionist.

When we delved into the problem, we advanced a new understanding. What was her boss's primary complaint? Veronica did not treat hard deadlines with sufficient seriousness. It was important for her to realize that although his view of her was inaccurate, it was not an un-fair impression. How so? "This work environment can be crazy and hec-tic, with constant deadline pressures," said Veronica. "I keep my wits about me by staying as calm as possible. I could see how I might seem too casual." But Veronica did not use this information to beat herself up. "I am certainly mindful of deadlines. If anything, I try too hard to be conscientious and responsible." The combination of intense pressure, and Veronica's effort to detach herself from the frenzy, did cause her to miss some deadlines. But she did not have to punish herself for her imperfections.

Veronica's insights led her to a wise remedy. She decided to assert herself to her boss. She told him, "I know I've been late on a few proj-ects, and I'm sorry. I am cognizant of deadlines, but I try to stay above the fray so I can concentrate and keep my work at the highest level pos-sible. Please don't think I am blasé about getting work done on time. I'll do better in the future."

Veronica's boss responded well to her honesty. She had corrected the misimpression that fueled his judgments and her insecurities. Veronica's communication was courageous and self-nurturing, but she would never have initiated the conversation if she hadn't already engaged in a courageous and self-nurturing analysis of her own thought distortions.

Consider these examples of how you can restructure negative thoughts about your work and career:

NEGATIVE THOUGHT: "I can't do this job."
RESTRUCTURED THOUGHT: "My work presents immense challenges,
                       and I do wonder whether I have
                       adequate training and experience to
                       handle them. But when I look into my
                       past, giving myself the benefit of the
                       doubt, I realize that I have risen to the
                       occasion in new and demanding work
                       situations. My learning curve may not be
                       steep, but it is steady. Once I grasp what's
                       expected, and become comfortable with
                       a new set of skills, I do a fine job. I also
                       realize that periods of self-doubt are
                       normal for me. When these insecurities

arise, I can say to myself, Big surprise!
That's just how my mind works."

NEGATIVE THOUGHT: "My colleague is much more skilled; I'll
never live up to her standards."

RESTRUCTURED THOUGHT: "My colleague is very bright, energetic,
and skillful. But if I stop viewing her
through the lens of my own anxieties, it's
clear that she's no more perfect than I
am. Just as I have certain deficits, so does
she. If I am fair, I realize that she has
strengths I lack, and I have strengths that
she lacks. Instead of framing my
relationship with her through
competitiveness, perhaps I can improve
my own skills by identifying her
strengths and emulating some of them,
to the best of my ability."

NEGATIVE THOUGHT: "I'll never have a career that gives me
meaning and joy."

RESTRUCTURED THOUGHT: "It's true that my current job yields no
meaning and little joy. But it's not
logical, or truthful, to assume that I can
never have a career that I love. No one is
stopping me from going back to school
and developing a set of skills for work
that would make me delighted to get up
in the morning. Yes, I'd have to work
part-time to support myself through
school, but with my goal firmly in mind,
it would be worth it. The problem now is
clear: every day on this job is like a
rebuke, a nasty message to myself that
says, This is all there is, and all there will
be. If I can rouse my fighting spirit, I can
reject that message! If I proceed with
patience and the utmost compassion for
myself, I can transform my work life."

Use cognitive restructuring to pick apart your self-denigrating assumptions, insecurities, unfounded fears, and worst-case scenarios. Rarely are we defeated by our competitors at work. As we strive for success and joy in our careers, it's usually our own thoughts that defeat us.

For instance: How often do we anxiously compare ourselves to fellow workers or people in our field? Whether we consistently judge ourselves as inferior or superior, we are still motivated by self-doubt. We need to reframe our whole tendency to compare ourselves with others, whether our efforts are characterized by self-deprecation, rivalry, envy, or egotism.

In my career as a clinician and researcher of mind-body medicine, I have been mentored by two leading lights in the field, Herbert Benson, M.D., head of Harvard's Division of Behavioral Medicine, where I continue to work, and Joan Borysenko, Ph.D., who left the division some years ago. Both Benson and Borysenko are renowned, not only for their expertise in the mind-body field but for their extraordinary abilities as public speakers, motivators, and teachers. Early in my career, I was awed by their abilities, which led me to think: *I'll never grab hold of an audience the way Herb and Joan do.* In my own estimation, I came up short, primarily because I harbored the mistaken belief that the only way I could captivate an audience would be to speak in the manner of Benson or Borysenko. As I matured, in work and in life, I realized that I could hold an audience without having to be like my charismatic mentors. I had to develop my own style and delivery, which was completely different, but also unique. I realized that I could celebrate their gifts and my own, at the same time.

Too often, we judge ourselves cruelly with these comparisons, as if someone else's talents eradicate our own. "So-and-so is such a tremendous speaker and I stink." "So-and-so is a fabulous writer; I'll never live up." "So-and-so is a dynamic corporate leader, I'll always be second-rung." It's better to question our beliefs about others regarding their talent and skill as compared to ours. We can emulate and learn from our role models, then move on to the challenge of cultivating our own strengths.

Women in the workplace *do* face discrimination on the basis of sex, and I'm not just referring to salary discrepancies or the glass ceiling. We are often hurt by the subtle favoritism of men, a real phenomenon that can prevent us from moving forward in our careers. But we must use cognitive restructuring to ferret out the truth: Are my male colleagues really being favored? If so, can I bring this to the attention of superiors through assertive communication? When you identify instances of unfairness, and action gets you nowhere, better to find another job than to remain the victim. On the other hand, cognitive work can help you determine whether your own mind is a more savage oppressor than your boss or institutional hierarchy. If so, you should expend more time and energy overthrowing the tyrant within.

The purpose of cognitive restructuring is to:

- Tell yourself the truth about your work-related stressors
- Reject self-negating thoughts
- Acknowledge your mistakes and imperfections with loving kindness
- Initiate needed changes through assertive action and communication
- Stop being the victim! Discard the notion that a hostile environment—even if it's one you can't change—has the power to destroy your capacity for joy at work. You have the choice either to adapt or leave.

Suzanne C. Ouellette, Ph.D., a psychologist at the City University of New York, has devoted her career to studying the personalities of people who stay strong, healthy, and happy in the world of work. She uses the term "hardiness" to define this personality type. Hardiness is actually three traits rolled into one: control, commitment, and challenge. The "three C's" refer to a sense of control over one's quality of life and health; a strong commitment to one's work, creative activities, or relationships; and a view of stress as a challenge rather than a threat. In a series of landmark studies at the University of Chicago, Ouellette followed nearly 700 workers undergoing the severe stress of corporate reorganization and downsizing. Some workers succumbed to the pressure by becoming distressed or physically ill, while others did not. The hardy workers, who resisted the damaging effects of work stress, displayed the "three C's" in abundance.

Ouellette is convinced that we can develop control, commitment, and challenge in our work lives. I agree wholeheartedly. Not only can we build the three C's, but doing so will reduce our risks of stress-related illness and enhance our capacity for joy at work. Ouellette's program is similar, in many respects, to my own. It centers on cognitive restructuring, decisive action, and self-improvement. Viewing stress as a challenge rather than a threat is the simplest, most powerful form of positive reframing. Let it become your mantra.

One way to embrace the three C's, says Ouellette, is to consider the dominant stressful situation in your life, past or present, and write down three ways it could be worse and three ways it could be better. Understanding how the situation could be worse gives you balance and perspective; understanding how it could be better underscores the ways you can take control and cultivate that sense of challenge. Next, imagine—and write down—specific steps you could take to bring about the better outcomes. This process is likely to trigger the part of your brain that searches for novel solutions.

Say, for example, that you didn't get the raise you feel you deserve. You're angry with your boss because you think he doesn't acknowledge your ability or hard work. As you spin out your worst-case fantasies, you imagine you've been demoted or fired. Now ask yourself what would have to be different in order for your boss to take such drastic measures. In all likelihood, while he may not appreciate your talents, he's not deliberately malicious. He is, however, very busy and often disorganized, so that he often doesn't have the time to review your work properly.

Ask yourself what steps you can take to improve your situation. Develop a strategy to improve communication between the two of you. For example, more frequent E-mails; regularly scheduled short meetings; memos to update him about your progress on various projects. When you take this kind of creative approach to problem solving, you can confront your reality with clearer, more accurate insights. Then you can view your situation as a challenge rather than as a threat.

Catharsis, Insight, Action: Nurture Emotions at Work

Jennie worked as an assistant to an entertainment lawyer, a middle-aged hard driver who kept her on her toes every hour of the day. When she began the job a year ago, Jennie was excited by the fast pace and the challenges. But she began feeling depressed after an accumulation of critical remarks by her boss. Ceaselessly hounded by one negative thought—"I'm worthless at work"—she began to feel demoralized, isolated, and uncertain about her future. Jennie had recently earned her law degree, and had seen her apprenticeship as a chance to learn and advance. The difficulties with her boss made her doubt her capacity to live out her dream of becoming an entertainment lawyer.

Many of us have such experiences on the job. We feel small, unimportant, or unrecognized. The power structure may be top-heavy with men, and the glass ceiling that looms above may seem utterly unbreakable. Our task is to find creative ways to overcome these obstacles. But before we abandon ship in a work situation where we feel stalled or disrespected, we should test whether we can use self-nurturance to strengthen ourselves.

After a few sessions with Jennie, it became apparent to me that she was chronically angry at her boss for his relentless criticism. But she was only dimly aware of that anger. Unrecognized anger clouds our vision, until we lose not only our perspective but our ability to take action on our own behalf. I encouraged Jennie to acknowledge that anger through a writing exercise. I told her to write out her deepest thoughts and feelings about her boss and his behavior. No inhibition, no stopping, no grammatical correctness, no calm reflection. Do this for 20 minutes over four days, I suggested, and notice the changes that take place.

Before doing this exercise, Jennie had begun to dread every workday. She'd slogged through her job in a haze of self-doubt, worrying about her productivity, anticipating the next unpleasant interaction with her boss. The anger exercise changed all that. She wrote, "I am sick and tired of his comments. He undermines me, then calls me 'honey,' then blasts my work. He taps right into my reservoir of self-doubt, the very thing I have been fighting all my life."

After doing the 20-minute writing process four days running, Jennie was suffused with energy and feeling. Her emotional stance changed from, "What have I done wrong?" to "How can he treat me this way?" It was a healthy transformation for Jennie, whose tendency had always been to shoulder blame. (For those of us who tend to blame others for our problems, "What have I done wrong?" might be an appropriate question. Not for Jennie.) Now Jennie was able to banish the false evidence she'd accumulated against herself and start collecting evidence that she was an effective worker. As it happened, there was abundant proof of her value to the firm, but she'd never given it much credence before.

Jennie had turned a corner, and then she found the following variety of self-nurturing ways to cope with her stress on the job.

- Shared notes on the boss with other colleagues
- Turned to empathetic friends on the job and finally confided her distress.
- Created a healthy distance between her and the boss, enough distance to be able to laugh about his behavior
- Observed how coworkers had developed skillful ways of handling his attempted manipulations, and began applying some of their tactics
- Found the courage, on occasion, to challenge the boss's unfairly critical comments directly, letting him know that she disagreed with his assessment and then walking away

While not a panacea for job stress, the emotional writing exercise often spurs a shift toward self-nurture, as it did for Jennie. Here are the seven steps you can follow for this exercise, including follow-up actions you can take on your own behalf.

- **Is there someone at work who causes you emotional suffering?**
- **If so, write your deepest thoughts and feelings about what they do or have done to cause you pain. Don't worry about sentence structure or good writing. Write the way painter Jackson Pollock attacked his canvas—with purpose and abandon.**
- **Do this exercise for 20 minutes every day for four days running.**
- **After the four days—but not before—read over what you've written. Notice changes in your writings from day to day in how you feel about your boss, supervisor, colleague, or coworker.**
- **Has your anger toward the person changed? Is it more or less intense? Have you come to understand the person better?**
- **Having worked through your anger, do you see the possibility of changing your relationship? What can you do to improve working relations? How would you like your boss/supervisor/ coworker to change his or her behavior toward you?**

- **Can you clearly imagine stating your need for respect, acceptance, or opportunity? If so, consider a shift from imagination to action: In the spirit of self-nurture, can you find the right time, place, and words to express your desire for a change? Can you do so with firmness but also with the same kind of respect you want from your counterpart? Can you model the very qualities you wish the other person would bring to your encounters?**

Be as honest as possible in your writing exercise. Don't express emotions you *think* you are supposed to express. In Jennie's case, she had to vent her anger toward herself before she could even uncover her anger toward her boss. If you find yourself expressing self-hatred on the page, keep writing—eventually that anger against yourself will move outward—toward someone who is inflicting harm or hurt on you. Many of my patients use writing to find and release their rage. Inevitably, as with Jennie, this emotional release makes them stronger—more able to channel their energies in constructive acts of self-assertion.

One of the best ways to nurture your emotional self on the job is to seek empathic coworkers who can listen and provide moral support. Jennie had neglected to seek that support because her emotional energies were so completely directed against herself. When she tentatively approached a fellow office assistant and broached the subject of their boss, he blurted out, "Oh, yeah. He's a little jerk." Jennie reacted with a wave of cathartic laughter, and her feelings about both her boss and herself began to change.

Be certain to confide in colleagues capable of empathy. If you find people who have had similar experiences with your boss, they can help you realize you're not crazy or incompetent. Best of all is finding a friend who not only validates your experiences, but who can also help you examine your *own* responses. A trusted person can help you see your part of the dance; that is, "We know about his or her baggage, but what could I be bringing to this encounter that is getting in our way?"

Not only can your work compatriots help you to reality-test, their moral support and friendship can ease the daily grind of a pressure-packed work environment. Many women silently bare their unhappiness at work, feeling they don't want to burden others. As a result, they feel alone even if pleasant people abound in their environment.

We're fortunate when we find friendly coworkers who not only listen and support, but who gently goad us to explore the tougher questions.

LABOR OF LOVE:
NURTURE SELF AND SPIRIT AT WORK

Meaning and purpose are existential vitamins; they keep us going beyond our normal limits of mental and physical energy. But even jobs we love can take a toll. This holds true particularly for women, who not only work their jobs as hard as their male counterparts, but often lopsidedly bear the burden of housework and child-rearing, even in these "enlightened" times. Meaning and purpose go a long way, but they don't enable us to leave our bodies. Philosophers, saints, and rock stars get exhausted just like the rest of us.

When our jobs are not labors of love, exhaustion and spiritual depletion frequently occur. In either case, nurturing self and spirit is the only antidote to job-related burnout. To accomplish this, ask yourself whether or not your work is a source of enjoyment and meaning. If your answer is no, then survival necessitates that you inject meaning and self-care into the crevices of your days. If your answer is yes, that is far from the end of the discussion. We burn out in jobs we love, too.

If your job lacks meaning and enjoyment, begin to question whether you want to remain full-time (or even part-time) in such a stultifying situation. When financial needs or motivations are paramount, try viewing the job you dislike for what it really is—a paycheck, a means to another end. This may help you break the cycle of feeling so bad about it. Meanwhile, take time to consider long-term alternative career plans. Visualize yourself doing the work you love, and you'll have the strength to endure and overcome short-term hindrances.

Joan, a fifty-three-year-old single woman, lived at home with her mother all her life. Joan was born with cerebral palsy, and though ambulatory, she suffers from a serious disturbance in her sense of balance. Her legs are weak with osteoarthritis due to a near-complete absence of cartilage in her joints. Joan's disabilities have not kept her from work; for years, she had a desk job in a local bank.

Eight years ago, Joan decided to enter social work school. She passionately embraced the idea of a job where she doled out guidance and support to people in need. Nothing, she thought, could make her happier. But her family, including her older sister, whom she adores, and her mother, with whom she has a difficult relationship, disapproved. They were convinced that Joan was risking her financial security by leaving her bank job. They worried that she wouldn't have enough money for retirement, and they pressured her to change course. In Joan's view, these concerns masked deeper ones. "They treated me as though I couldn't do anything," she said. "My family thinks of me as the baby sister. I have a feeling they don't want me to grow." Joan realized what she was up against, but refused to let it stop her. "This is my life, and I have a right to make these decisions," was her clarion call. She brooked her family's disfavor and enrolled in social work school. Three years later, she graduated with her bachelor's degree. "Graduation day was the happiest day of my life," she said. "It had taken me thirty years to find out what I wanted to do, but I did it."

Her family did not celebrate Joan's triumph, but that has not prevented her from moving forward. She found a part-time job working with the elderly at the local Council on Aging. Today, Joan is committed to three goals: finding a full-time social work position; getting her master's degree; and moving out of her mother's house. Joan believes that her family has gotten used to her dependence, and so has she. While the road ahead is long and tough, she fully expects to win her independence—to live on her own and do work she loves and is proud of.

"I'm not a little kid anymore," she says. "I need to take care of myself. I want to grow and experience new things, as much as I can and to the fullest extent of my talents."

Like Joan, we need to find a way to view our problems—internal or external, mental or physical, practical or financial—as hard challenges that rouse the best in us, rather than impenetrable walls we might never scale. We cultivate enormous strength as long as we feel passionately about the goal we're working toward—a career that excites us, stirs our creativity, engages our talents, and gives us a powerful raison d'être.

There are times in our lives, of course, when our jobs don't offer the meaning, purpose, and joy we seek. Sometimes, we keep these jobs because we have to—money is short, time is short, and we're still working on long-range plans. In the meantime, we can inject meaning and self-care into our days by stoking our commitment to self-nurture at work. Here are some practical strategies you can undertake *now*:

- **Create Your Work Space.** Even if only a cubicle, make your work space your own, with pictures, paintings, books, or other artifacts that generate a sense of calm, remind you of the world outside work, or remind you that you belong where you are. The pictures can be family shots (but don't have to be) or landscapes, faces, movie stills from your favorite films, the work of the world's great photographers. Bring healthy snacks, savory coffees, or calming herb teas to keep in your desk and prepare during breaks when you need nourishment or relaxation. Buy yourself a special mug. If certain aromas create a pleasurable atmosphere, wear that perfume or bring that scent in a bottle to your work space. In your selection of work clothes or decorative touches for your space, pay attention to colors that evoke moods of serenity or confidence. My desk is covered with pictures of Dave and Sarah, as well as lots of small ceramic penguins, because all my friends know I collect penguins.
- **Use Breaks to Revitalize.** Use your breaks as time for eliciting the relaxation response or for reading. Try focused daydreaming instead of spacing out. Bring your Walkman to work and select soul-satisfying tapes or CDs to hear on breaks or while you work, if that's possible. Get outside as often as possible; being stuck in an office without moving your body for endless hours leads to mind-body disconnection. Simple walking is often enough to remind us that we reside in our bodies.
- **Set Priorities.** Stress experts have long counseled that we make concerted efforts on the job to list priorities: tease out the tasks that need doing right away, and concentrate on them. The other tasks may beckon, attached as they are to some goal, or to someone who wants something right now. But if we focus, we'll know which work assignment is top priority and which supervisors really need immediate results. It's also a good idea to reward yourself with the "fun" stuff after doing the "boring" stuff. For instance, the aspect of my work I love most is working in groups or individual sessions with my patients. But as a health psychologist in a hospital-based program packed with clients, I must spend considerable time in my office taking care of administrative tasks. One of the tasks I hate is updating charts on my patients; for me the process is dreadfully dull. One office task I enjoy is returning phone calls to pa-

tients and colleagues. So I limit myself to an hour of charting and reward myself with an hour of phone calls. It breaks up the day into alternating segments of necessary tasks and pleasurable contacts, and it helps me maintain my enthusiasm and energy.

- **Seek Support from Friends.** Find people on the job who share some of your values, perspectives on work, and sense of humor. If this sounds simplistic, think again. I've found that many overextended women overlook people in their midst who could be supportive work friends. When your world is chaotic, making contact can seem like just one more chore. But taking time to slow down and consider who we want to relax with and making the extra bit of effort required can yield huge benefits. Perhaps we can apply a litmus question: Which lunch partner is likely to make me laugh?

The Job/Family/Self Equation: Making It Work

Working mothers face a whole other set of complex challenges to their ability to nurture self and spirit. Perhaps my own experience as a mother with time-consuming professional demands will be instructive. My focus is to ensure that I have time to get my work done, be with my husband and daughter, get enough rest and exercise, and still nurture myself with pleasurable activities. In most respects I'm probably no different from most working Moms, except that I've made self-nurture a major priority, and I've tried to plan my weeks and months in advance to make certain I meet these goals. (Also, I'm really fortunate that I've been able to modify my work schedule to best meet my needs.)

Here's what I mean. On Sundays, I make a huge meal—a big pot of chicken soup or a turkey or a large roast chicken—that provides leftovers for at least two or three days during the week. On weeknights I'll prepare fresh vegetables and other side dishes to perk up the leftovers, but that still cuts my cooking time dramatically. When we have Chinese take-out, we order huge quantities so that we have ample leftovers. I'm fortunate as I am able to work at home two days a week. I have flexibility, so I work at my office from 10:00 A.M. to 6:00 P.M. the other days. My husband and I have purposely staggered our work schedules, so he's gone from 7:00 A.M. to 4:00 P.M. This enables me to spend time every morning with my daughter Sarah; until 9:00 A.M., we hang out, talk, play games, snuggle. On this schedule I also miss rush-hour traffic, which saves a great deal of time, and I use the morning commute to plan work activities and the evening commute to plan family activities. My husband gets quality time with Sarah in the late afternoon before I return home.

I know that the only way I'm going to grab enough time with my husband and daughter, and still find opportunities to nurture myself (for me, by reading the paper, taking hot baths, and going out with friends), is to devise new time-saving strategies constantly. I keep lists of every item I need at the convenience drug store so I make as few trips as possible. I go to superstores where I buy huge quantities of household products—many months' worth of paper towels, napkins, Q-tips, etc. I keep lists of birthday and Christmas gifts I need to get long in advance so I can do my gift-buying in the fewest number of excursions. I sometimes rent videos for my daughter so she is occupied, and far less miserable, when I must return phone calls in the evening.

I don't cut corners on sleep time, since I'm unbearably cranky when I don't get my eight hours. But I choose a form of exercise that also allows me to self-nurture with my loved ones. I take long walks and hikes with my husband and daughter on the weekends and some weeknights, and just with my husband once or twice during the week while Sarah is at day care. Being outdoors and moving my limbs is wonderful for my mind-body state. It grants me an opportunity to teach my daughter about mindfulness; we laugh, sing, and kick stones while I encourage her to take in the sights, sounds, and smells. My husband and I surely benefit from the time to simply be together, in silence or in conversations about what matters most to us at the time.

I offer my strategies not as a perfect model—you should see how messy my house often is—but as an example of how the effort of such planning can pay off. There is no simple route to managing the work/family/time dilemma, but we can make things easier by bringing every ounce of intelligence and creativity to the task. Make certain, however, that your primary goals are threefold, not twofold. If you limit yourself to getting work done and finding time with family, you can easily forget about yourself. One reason I have the energy to live my life with zest is because I *do* self-nurture, as much as possible, knowing that the time spent on myself is also crucial for my work and my family.

You might ask what a spiritual perspective at work could possibly mean. Anything you do to inject pleasure and meaning into your work can resonate on deeper levels. But there are other spiritual questions about work, and even tentative answers can yield an ineffable sense of the sacred in our daily activity. What is my purpose here? What can I learn at work? What can I contribute? I may not love every aspect of my job, but can I find compensatory pleasure in it? Pockets of purpose, places where I can make a difference? Opportunities to test my talents, raise my sights, or explore creative abilities? If you can't answer yes to any one of these questions, formulate a sensible long-range plan for moving on.

Perhaps your work tasks themselves lack intrinsic creative potential or value to others. But you may be able to find meaning in your relations with others at work. For instance, when it comes to social support, we often have a blinkered view: What can I get from So-and-so? Who can meet my needs? These are sound questions, and I've encouraged you to ask them. But social support works two ways; if we view ourselves only as receivers, the quality of our support is impoverished. Our work lives are enriched when we not only *get* support but *offer* support to people we care about. If a coworker is suffering ill-treatment from your employer, a suffering you have also known, then listening to her is more than a gift you bestow—it's a gift you receive in kind. Sharing the experience creates a bond of understanding that eases the isolation, anger, or self-doubt you both experience. Those of us in the helping professions have that pleasure built into our work, but it's a viable path toward spiritual sustenance for everyone who works.

When I say "spiritual," I refer to moving beyond the separate self, if only momentarily, to come in contact with spirit—whatever that means in your belief system. Much has been written about the spiritual aspects of service, be it formal helping or daily acts of kindness. When we reach out to help, we reach beyond the self. People who devote their lives to service tell us that their work leads to in ineffable "connection to something larger than ourselves." In their book about service and spirituality, *How Can I Help?*, Ram Dass and Paul Gorman use the term "Unity" to describe that sense of absolute connectedness. "Unity will finally mean something to us only as the felt truth of direct experience," write Ram Dass and Gorman. "We find it in the power and beauty of a single, simple caring act." Simple caring acts in the workplace can transform our relationship not only to our colleagues but to work itself.

Finally, I suggest certain affirmations about work that you can use in your relaxation or meditation practices. You can even repeat affirmations to yourself in the midst of difficult work situations, or during short breaks or mini-relaxation exercises. These are especially effective when things go badly, when obligations overwhelm, or you doubt your skills and creativity.

"I am not my job."
"I am entitled to make mistakes."
"I have the strength and skill to succeed."
"I have a right to fairness."
"My creativity knows no bounds."
"Stillness in body and mind."
"Letting go of tension and anxiety . . ."
"I embrace the challenge."

Use these affirmations or write your own. Keep them straight and simple; high-flown philosophy rarely translates to our unconscious mind.

Work is an essential part of who we are, yet we are not our jobs. Nonetheless, there are times when we forget that we're bigger than our jobs. As long as we nurture other facets of ourselves—our humor, capacity for play, family lives, friendships, and spirituality—the demands of work will never threaten to completely overtake our lives and steal our lightness of being.

9

THE FAITH FACTOR:

OUR SINGULAR SPIRITUALITY

The force that inspires the heart to believe is not identical with the impulse that stimulates the mind to reason. . . . It is faith from which we draw the sweetness of life, the taste of the sacred, the joy of the imperishably dear. It is faith that offers us a share in eternity. It is faith in which the great things occur.
—Abraham Joshua Heschel

FOR MOST OF US, the word nurture, from the Latin *nutritus* for "nourish," conjures images of taking care of others with lovingly prepared food, emotional support, protective warmth, practical help, and wise teachings. In self-nurture, we offer ourselves these same gifts, and more, as a daily practice. But there is another form of "nourishment" that I haven't mentioned as a formal aspect of self-nurture—spirituality. For we can nourish ourselves with spiritual experiences through prayer or other practices, whether we define that reality as God's love, the love of another person, a higher power, an incarnate force, or Nature with a capital *N*.

The metaphor of spirituality as nourishment is no intellectual fancy. We can repress our need for spirit, and as a result, we can be starved of spirit, suffering varieties of "malnourishment"—confusion, boredom, disconnectedness. Filling our need for spiritual illumination can heal these disturbing maladies of the soul. The key is that we cultivate a *self-nurturing spirituality.*

What is a self-nurturing spirituality? One in which our search for meaning and purpose is consciously woven into our daily lives, rather than relegated to religious holiday reflections or New Year's resolutions.

It's one in which we come to terms with our religious background, ferreting out, as best we can, our own core beliefs about God or spirit. One in which we are, finally, beholden only to ourselves when it comes to our ultimate decisions about faith and how we practice it. One in which our understanding of God or spirit, however defined, imbues us with a boundless compassion rather than heartless judgments of both ourselves and others. One in which our faith is less a reflection of childhood magical thinking than a mature awareness of our connectedness with others, nature, and the universe.

In my experience with women in the grip of emotional or physical suffering, a self-nurturing spirituality is no easy prescription. On some religious or cosmic plane, we may feel as though God or spirit has abandoned us. We may attribute our unworthiness to different factors—we don't believe strongly enough, we aren't religious enough, we haven't prayed enough, or we've sinned far too much. Some of us were alienated from our religious training, and then lost faith in *any* spiritual construct, no matter how different from the long-discarded precepts of our childhood religion. In my view, those of us without spiritual grounding—who are confused, pessimistic, or cynical, lacking faith in ourselves and our world—may be stuck precisely because we can't seek comfort from a spiritual framework that is truly self-nurturing.

My parents were both raised in Jewish homes, but I received a minimum of formal religious training. Yet I feel Jewish, because I was exposed to Jewish cultural influences, and I respect Jewish history and culture. Still, having had so little experience with Jewish rituals of prayer and observance, I don't really relate to these religious beliefs. Even so, whenever I'm faced with a health crisis, I suddenly find myself reaching toward a higher power.

Over a year ago, as the New Year approached, I began to experience abdominal pain, bloating, and back pain. Once I recognized this particular constellation of symptoms, I was seized by fear. I knew they could be early signs of ovarian cancer. I went straight to my internist, who echoed my concerns (an echo I didn't want to hear), and immediately ordered an ultrasound and blood tests for tumor markers. Before I had the ultrasound, I engaged in a classic form of bargaining: "God, if all these tests are negative and I don't have cancer, I promise to take better care of myself. I'm going to sleep more, eat better, exercise regularly, and do whatever I can to keep such a terrible event from coming to pass."

When the ultrasound revealed no tumor, I breathed that familiar sigh of relief, the kind that clears the mind and body of all anxiety—and all promises, too. I'd made such deals before, and I hadn't always kept up my end of the bargain once I'd been "let off the hook." This time, I made a better effort. I've seen too many women, dear friends and patients, die of breast or ovarian cancer.

Such moments prompt us to conduct inventories of our behavior, but they also prompt us to examine our spiritual beliefs. Does God work that way? Can we bargain with our higher power? I don't know, but the notion that God or spirit "wants" us to take good care of ourselves strikes a chord with me. (The part I wonder about is whether we're rewarded or punished with good or bad health.) When we make a pact with ourselves to tend to our physical and emotional well-being, we might also consider it a pact with a higher power, even if it's only our highest self.

In the decade I've been directing mind-body programs, I have taught my patients how to use prayer as one form of meditation, but I have not emphasized the broader role of spirituality in women's health and well-being. Recently, this has changed. I've begun to incorporate spiritual coping in my work with women, whether they're confronting cancer, menopause, pelvic pain, depression, infertility, divorce, or any other crisis. One reason for the change is the exciting work being carried out here in the Mind/Body Medical Institute, under the direction of Herbert Benson, a world-renowned leader in spirituality and health. Dr. Benson spearheads major conferences and research projects on the mind-body-spirit connection, and he's written a compelling overview of the field, *Timeless Healing.* The other reason is that so many patients passionately wish to incorporate spirituality into their healing process. Whether they want to integrate their religious beliefs with mind-body practices, or simply yearn for spiritual comfort or meaning as they endure an illness, they've let me know that this dimension is essential to them.

Women dealing with infertility, in particular, have often sought religious or spiritual comfort as they undergo the rigors of medical treatments, rising hopes, and serial bouts of sorrow. Some wish to rebuild their shattered faith, others are searching for a faith they've never had, while still others are seeking answers to difficult spiritual questions. To meet this need, I found a collaborator, Barbara Nielsen, who is both an Episcopal minister and a therapist. Barbara has carried out a pilot study with a group of twelve infertility patients, and she now attends many sessions of our infertility program. She teaches our participants about spiritual coping—how they can nourish their singular spirituality as they endure the emotional roller-coaster ride of infertility and its treatment.

Together, Barbara and I have tried to offer women a framework for a self-nurturing spirituality. She's conducted her own research on the link between religious beliefs and women's self-esteem. "Our self-understanding," says Barbara, "is based on entering a relationship with a God who expects us to be ourselves, to manifest our light and let it shine. There is a passage in the Beatitudes that translates as, 'Don't hide your light under a bushel.' I think that is a real command to all people not to take a secondary role in life, but to get out there, be who you are, and do what you love."

Remember, as you proceed with spiritual self-nurture, that spirituality and religiosity are not synonymous. In some women's lives, they overlap completely: their religious life *is* their spiritual life. Others have a rich spiritual life with few or no ties to organized religion. I believe you should define your own spirituality in the depths of your heart and mind, not according to any orthodoxy, whether from the Old World or the New Age.

NURTURE THE BODY: RELAXATION AND PRAYER

In the late 1960s and early 1970s, Herbert Benson documented the profound physiological changes—reduced blood pressure, heart rate, oxygen consumption, and skin conductance, among others—that occurred among practitioners of transcendental meditation when they dropped into deep meditation. He dubbed this altered psychophysical state the "relaxation response," and continued to investigate whether other, related practices would produce similar results. One such practice was prayer. "To be sure that modern religious practices could evoke the relaxation response, we brought into our laboratory people who regularly prayed," writes Benson. "We found that repetitive prayer—in Judaism, a *davening*-type prayer; in Catholicism, a rosary-type prayer; and in Protestantism, a "centering" prayer—produced the same physiological changes that we had originally noted in transcendental meditation. We now recommend that our religious patients consider using such prayer when they elicit the relaxation response and that nonreligious patients use any sound, word, or phrase with which they feel comfortable."

The benefits of prayer may go beyond affecting the vital signs. People may indeed experience improved health or recovery from illness. "More than 130 controlled laboratory studies show, in general, that prayer or a prayerlike state of compassion, empathy, and love can bring about healthful changes in many types of living things, from humans to bacteria," writes physician and prayer expert Larry Dossey in *Prayer Is Good Medicine.* "This does not mean that prayer always works, any more than drugs and surgery always work, but that, statistically speaking, prayer is effective."

And it is not just prayer by itself that may support the healing process. Epidemiologist Jeffrey Levin of Eastern Virginia Medical School, possibly the world expert on spirituality and health, has uncovered more than 250 published studies on the largely beneficial health effects of religious or spiritual practice. Levin's work does not explain how spiritual involvement promotes health. But Levin offers a number of theories, including behavioral factors (i.e., religious observance may be linked to less smoking or alcohol); social support (i.e., strong ties with a community of observers); psychological uplift (i.e., relief of anxiety and depression that, in turn, bolsters our biological systems); or, most controversially, the divine intervention of a spiritual entity or energy. Mainstream science may never develop instruments that can quantify divine intervention, though some of the prayer research cited by Larry Dossey suggests that prayer can have effects outside the body. Namely, several studies on "intercessory" prayer—praying for others—have shown that prayed-for people experience better health outcomes than members of a control group who are not prayed for.

Whatever our beliefs, the research on spiritual practices and health can no longer be ignored. Even if the benefits are strictly social and psychological, that should be enough for us to consider cultivating a self-nurturing spirituality that can, potentially, enhance our physical as well as emotional health.

Self-Nurturing Prayer

Harriet's ritual before going to sleep and upon awakening was the same every day: She fingered her rosary beads while saying Hail Mary's. Then she asked God for a full recovery from breast cancer.

Harriet had never been a devout Catholic, and in most ways her diagnosis of invasive cancer had not caused a complete turnabout in her religious observance. She did start attending church a bit more regularly, but the primary change was that her previous intermittent praying—"I'd say a Hail Mary a few times when something really bad happened"—became a highly ritualized daily practice. Harriet likened the effect of her diagnosis to an earthquake, and it made her question both her reason for being and her relationship to God. "I think I found my way back to the part of religious belief that meant something to me as a child," she said. "The simple prayerful attitude I had when I would say a Hail Mary" was the essence of what was right about Catholicism for me. That direct relationship with God, without the other trappings. When I was so afraid, especially during the chemo period, I found myself going right back there."

Harriet had no illusions that her prayers would surely prevent her breast cancer from recurring. Nevertheless, she was comforted by the ritual. Her prayers seemed to center and strengthen her. "I felt as if He had put some steel in my backbone."

Four years after her surgery, and an arduous year of chemotherapy treatments with several bouts of severe infection, Harriet is cancer-free and in excellent health. Has she continued to pray? Yes, she told me, but not every day. Still, she prays with more regularity—and conviction—than she did prior to her chemotherapy, and she insists that she's fashioned a vastly richer religious life than she ever experienced in her "B.C." (before cancer) life.

Harriet alluded to the fact that her B.C. religious life was at best ambivalent, because there were aspects of Catholicism, in terms of theology and ritual, that turned her off. Like many baby boomers, she recovered her religiosity after confronting a harrowing life crisis, and she did so by selectively seizing on elements of the religious traditions of her childhood that she could relate to. She rejected the all-or-nothing position of religious orthodoxy that had previously prevented her from finding an authentic and livable way of being a Catholic.

I don't present Harriet's story as a brief against religious orthodoxy. Many people thrive psychologically, morally, and spiritually by hewing as closely as possible to their religious traditions. My point here is that a self-nurturing spirituality is one most consonant with your individual philosophy, emotional life, and personality—one that meets your needs, rouses your compassion, and provides that "connection to something larger than yourself."

That said, certain types of prayer—regardless of the organized tradition from which they stem—tend to yield certain emotional and physiologic results. While there is no "right" way to pray, you can choose approaches to prayer that are congruent with your personality, philosophy, and needs at a particular time. Larry Dossey makes the point that some of us are "prayer dropouts" because our personalities never meshed with the prayer rituals of the organized religion in which we were raised. The prayer dropouts among us may benefit from compassionate flexibility, allowing ourselves to experiment until we find a way of praying that works for us, rather than rejecting prayer altogether.

Certainly, there are many types of prayer. But as you develop your prayer practice, consider the two broad styles typically labeled "directed" and "nondirected." The former refers to prayer in which you ask God, the universe, or a spiritual presence to bring about a specific outcome. The latter refers to a nonspecific approach in which you hold no outcome in heart and mind. In his book *Healing Words*, Larry Dossey dubs them the "make it happen" versus "let it be" approaches, respectively. In "make it happen," you beseech the higher power to intercede, to solve a particular problem, cure an illness, or relieve emotional suffering. In "let it be," you praise your deity or spiritual reality and pray only for the highest good—whatever that may be. This stance of surrender may be summed up as "thy will be done."

Dossey says that outgoing personalities usually prefer directed "make it happen" prayer, while introverts prefer nondirected "let it be" prayer. He cites studies suggesting that both types of prayer may be effective in bringing about particular outcomes in laboratory studies (such as a change of bacterial growth patterns in a Petri dish); there is little reason to pick one over the other because it is more likely to "work." We should choose a style of prayer that feels right for us.

For instance, both Dr. Benson's research and my own clinical experience suggest that nondirected "let it be" prayer—associated with a quiet, passive, reflective state of mind and body—is more likely to evoke the relaxation response. Beseeching, "make it happen" prayer won't always elicit the relaxation response, but it will surely rouse our emotions. Barbara Nielsen sees value in this unreserved petitionary prayer, and she encourages patients to "ask, plead, beg, scream, and yell" for what they want, whether it is pain relief, a pregnancy, the energy to function in everyday life, or a cancer remission. In Barbara's view, we should no more inhibit our true emotions in our relationship with God than in our relationships with loved ones.

Thus, if you wish to cultivate a relaxed, peaceful, accepting state of mind and body, I suggest nondirected prayer. You do so by adopting a passive meditative state, with awareness focused on the breath, and the repetition of a prayer word or phrase from a tradition in which you believe (See prayer guidelines in chapter 2). If you are brimming over with anxiety, rage, sorrow, or grief, you may find it helpful to express such strong feeling in prayer, following Barbara Nielsen's suggestion for petitionary prayer.

Barbara also recommends a combination of directed and nondirected prayer, a potentially powerful experience in which you freely petition your higher power for a specific outcome ("make it happen"), then adopt a stance of surrender ("let it be"). To illustrate the phases of this prayer process, she draws an X on a piece of paper. "The top part of the X represents prayers of asking—sending your petitions to God. The center of the X is the stillness into which you fall after you're done asking. The bottom of the X is the deep meditative state of listening." While Barbara encourages this "asking and listening," she also suggests that the prayer close with the ultimate invocation of "let it be": "Thy will be done, not mine."

This process enables you to express your wishes, which may be emotionally stirring, before falling into stillness and then a deep listening in which we accept our lack of control over every outcome. "Thy will be done, not mine" saves us from the illusion that we can press our higher power into meeting all our needs, and it saves us from the delusion that when things don't work out, it is because we did not pray correctly. "Thy will be done" recognizes, too, that the highest good may come from an outcome that differs from the one we so strenuously seek. I think of many infertility patients who have prayed unsuccessfully for a pregnancy, yet who went on to adopt a baby who became a beloved child.

One woman, who eventually adopted a boy from the Philippines, said to me, "I know this will sound weird, but I am so glad I did not have a biological child. Because I have the child I was supposed to have. Jonathan is the person who was supposed to be in our home."

Prayer does not always come easily, especially for those of us who feel disconnected from or uncertain about the religious traditions of our family of origin. If we wish to pray, we may need to develop our own rituals. Barbara Nielsen has an enormously helpful way of turning secular meditation into spiritual contemplation or prayer. Here is Barbara's approach, as she described it to me:

> I suggest to women in our groups that we focus on deep muscle relaxation and stilling of the mind. Now for a spiritual person that's not enough. We have to go more deeply into meditation. We've learned from our Buddhist sisters and brothers what it means to connect with God in the stillness. We need to get fully into stillness to create that kind of connection, one that allows us to be present with our guidance. For example, when a woman [with infertility, or any physical condition] is trying to make up her mind about what to say or do, what tests to take or not, she can go into that deep part of the relationship between herself and God; she can ask those questions in prayer and get an answer as she listens in meditation. Asking and listening, asking and listening.

To Each Her Own:
Nurture the Mind

How do we choose to believe? The word *choose* is vital, because our religious training often prods us to either accept the tenets and practices of our creed or not, and beyond this fork in the road there's no room for choice. This rigidity not only breeds prayer dropouts, it breeds religious dropouts who lose interest in any kind of spiritual life. It also breeds devout believers, but some of them suffer needlessly because they adopt practices and beliefs inconsistent with their true selves. I mean this less as a criticism of organized religion than a realistic recognition that many women can't swallow whole the religious doctrines of their childhood.

Cognitive restructuring can be enormously healing for spiritual dropouts, or for those believers who saddle themselves with religious dogma that causes more pain than enlightenment. Does a particular religious/spiritual belief or tenet promote feelings of worthlessness, inadequacy, or shame? (I'm not talking about healthy guilt—the basis for a moral conscience. I'm talking about gratuitous self-loathing.) If so, you need to subject this belief or tenet to the four questions of cognitive restructuring. In essence, you can put your religious or spiritual ideas to the test, and if you find them unrealistic and/or harmful to your emotional well-being, you can replace them with beliefs that you find both more truthful and compassionate.

Helen and her husband attended one of my weekend infertility workshops because they'd been trying to get pregnant for five years. Their lack of success had left them both feeling disheartened and confused. Helen's doctors could find no medical reason for her infertility, but Helen was convinced she knew why all their efforts had failed. She wept openly as she talked about the two abortions she'd undergone years earlier. A practicing Catholic who attended church every Sunday, she was sure that her inability to conceive was divine punishment for her "sins." When Helen applied cognitive restructuring, she realized that in her heart she believed in a merciful God, not one who would visit this kind of suffering upon her. Helen freed herself not from religion but from the part of religious dogma that caused gratuitous pain, the part that was not truly consistent with her bedrock beliefs.

Two months after the workshop, Helen called to tell me she was pregnant, and she has since given birth to a beautiful little boy. I can't help but wonder if there is some connection between her reexamination of her beliefs and her pregnancy.

Another case in point: One of my patients, Janice, had endured five miscarriages. Recurrent miscarriage is one of the most horrendous problems any woman can face. The death of a hoped-for child in utero is as real as any other death, and as the losses accumulate the grief can seem intolerable. Janice's anguish was exacerbated by her negative thought, "God is making me miscarry because I haven't suffered enough in my life."

As part of restructuring, I told Janice bluntly what I believed was the logical extension of her thought: "You're saying that God is causing the death of your babies." "No!" she protested, even as it dawned on her that this *was* the misguided logic at the core of her negative thought. Looked at from this perspective, Janice was horrified: the God she worshipped in her heart would not destroy a child as a way to punish a prospective mother. She began to question other assumptions, including her thought, "I haven't suffered enough." Was there something about her past and personality that made her feel she deserved an even bigger slice of tragedy? As Janice delved more deeply, she found the religious roots of her harsh views of herself and her God. Her religious training had taught her that God *could* be punitive in this way. Not only was she able to restructure her negative thoughts, Janice rebuilt her religious beliefs on a foundation of self-regard rather than self-punishment.

I tell patients like Janice that their restructuring is not a rejection of their God or religion. Rather, it enables them to refine their faith so it is compatible with their bedrock beliefs, and consonant with their essential selves. Moreover, a self-nurturing spirituality implies belief in a higher power (no matter how that power is understood) of compassion and forgiveness. I've worked with women who remained convinced that they deserve divine punishment for their transgressions—even after we practiced cognitive restructuring. I never try to talk these patients out of their convictions, but I encourage them to keep asking deeper questions, such as: Why do you need to suffer? What constitutes enough suffering? Can you acknowledge your transgressions and yet make peace with a compassionate deity? If you feel your God is a punishing one, can you explore whether your family, or others in your past, have inculcated you with feelings of shame and worthlessness?

Here are some other common negative thoughts associated with religious/spiritual life:

God is punishing me with illness because I've been too
   promiscuous.
God is punishing me with infertility because I had an abortion.
I have no faith because I lost a loved one, and I can't understand
   how any God could do that.
I have no spirituality because I hated the enforced religion of my
   childhood.
God wants me to suffer in this marriage because I've mistreated my
   spouse.

God made me terminally ill because I never believed or practiced
   my religion as I should have.
I must live a perfect life in order to deserve God's love.

Most people who read this list react swiftly: What a harsh, punitive
God! Close study of all the major religions—including Christianity,
Catholicism, Judaism, Islam, and Buddhism—reveals a compassionate
deity at the heart of their theology. Of course, we can also find images of
a punitive God, but each of us has to resolve such contradictions for
herself, which leads us right back to this question: *What do we choose to
believe?*

Here are two examples of how you can restructure negative spiritual
thoughts:

NEGATIVE THOUGHT: "I have no spirituality because I hated the
                         enforced religion of my childhood."
RESTRUCTURED THOUGHT: "It is true that I hated the enforced
                         religion of my childhood. But if I
                         honestly evaluate my thoughts and
                         feelings, I have to admit that I've thrown
                         out the baby with the bathwater. I was so
                         angry about the guilt my religion
                         induced in me that I rejected anything to
                         do with God. I'm now mature enough to
                         recognize that I don't have to remain
                         allergic to spirituality, as long as I can
                         reawaken aspects of faith that are
                         meaningful to me, that support my
                         intellectual and emotional well-being,
                         and that of my family and community. I
                         can return to rituals that I find moving; I
                         can even create my own rituals. In short,
                         I now realize that I can have a spiritual
                         life of my own that also draws from my
                         tradition."

NEGATIVE THOUGHT: "I have no faith because I lost a loved one,
                         and I can't understand how any God
                         could do that."

RESTRUCTURED THOUGHT: "I realize that my thought is based on the assumption that God is either uncaring, unconcerned, or actively involved in bringing about a tragedy. When I examine this thought, I realize it derives from my religious training, which taught that God rewards and punishes. But when I apply logic, I realize that everyone gets sick and everyone dies, no matter how good or bad. Perhaps God does not intervene in such simple ways, and perhaps I can transform my religious and spiritual beliefs to acknowledge a compassionate deity to whom I can turn for strength and wisdom, not for guarantees of longevity or immortality for myself or my loved ones."

Rabbi Harold Kushner is famous for *When Bad Things Happen to Good People*, a best-selling book that appeals to all faiths with its message that a God of love does not intervene to punish our every transgression or reward our every good deed with glorious gifts. If that were so, no "bad" person would ever get away with misdeeds, and no "good" person would ever be struck with illness or beset by tragedy. We know the world does not work that way. In his latest book, *How Good Do We Have to Be?*, Kushner helps us embrace a mature religious view:

God does not stop loving us every time we do something wrong, and neither should we stop loving ourselves and each other for being less than perfect. If religious teachers tell us otherwise, that is bad religion. If our parents responded to our misbehavior by withdrawing their love, that was a bad response by people who may otherwise have been good parents.

Kushner embraces a religion of compassion without rejecting the role of religion in shaping our moral conscience: "Religion condemns wrongdoing. It takes us to task for lying and hurting people. But religion also tries to wash us clean of disappointments in ourselves, with the liberating message that God finds us worthy of His love." Some of you will wish to substitute some other word for "God." Regardless of your concept of a deity or spiritual force, it is possible to stoke a self-nurturing spirituality, guided simply by what the Tibetan Dalai Lama calls "a policy of kindness." Kindness toward yourself and others can be the fount of your spiritual life.

REACHING OUT, LETTING GO: NURTURE THE EMOTIONS

A book edited by the former *New York Times* science writer Daniel Goleman, *Healing Emotions*, consists of conversations between the Dalai Lama and several experts in mind-body health. In one exchange with Jon Kabat-Zinn, the Dalai Lama addressed the links between emotions and self-esteem:

> DALAI LAMA: I am trying to trace the etiology [of low self-esteem], the natural causal links leading to this. To trace this, we note there is a sense of self that wishes for one's own happiness, and then the low self-esteem and self-deprecation come in. But underlying this, might there not already be compassion toward oneself on a deeper level? In that case, the low self-esteem is a distortion on a more superficial level, whereas underlying that is a sense of appropriate self-love.

> JON KABAT-ZINN: I think that's true, but if you can't get in touch with that sense of self-love then you feel cut off and alone.

> DALAI LAMA: If there is no genuine sense of love underlying all that emotion, then even if others praise you, you are not affected by that praise. When others praise a person with low self-esteem, he or she says they're wrong. The method Dan Brown described about affirmations to counter negative feelings was almost like reminding the patients of their own value. . . . But unless one assumes there is some kind of self-love underlying their emotion, it would be difficult to understand; there would be no motivation.

> JON KABAT-ZINN: I think there are deep reservoirs of love underlying all human beings.

DALAI LAMA: Oh, yes. I believe that's human nature. So long as one is a human being, that self-love should be there.

How do we unearth the self-love "underlying all that emotion"? The Dalai Lama spoke about positive affirmations that remind people of their own value—a form of spiritual self-nurture. A variety of psycho-spiritual approaches and practices help us move through layers of emotion to get to the self-love that both Kabat-Zinn and the Dalai Lama maintain *is there*.

I've been influenced by my work with Barbara Nielsen in developing a set of four ways to nurture the emotions through spiritually enlightening practice: nonidentification; reaching out; letting go; and the spirit of writing.

Nonidentification

This approach can be summed up in the phrase, "We have emotions, but we are not our emotions." This is consistent with many religious disciplines, but is most fully developed in Buddhism. We all tend to identify our entire selfhood with our emotions—as if we *are* the anger we feel at our forgetful husband, we *are* the sorrow we feel when a parent dies, we *are* the fear we feel when diagnosed with breast or ovarian cancer. We forget that such emotions are fleeting mind-states, not the sum-and-substance of our being. That does *not* mean that emotions are insubstantial, or to be repressed or ignored. They are an essential part of our selfhood, but they are not our *selves*.

Barbara Nielsen sums up this wisdom like this: "We have emotions but we're not our emotions; we have a body but we're not our body; we have a spirit and we *are* spirit." This awareness prevents us from identifying with our transient emotions, similar to meditation, where we watch the flow of thoughts and feelings rather than attach ourselves to them. When we accomplish this, our selfhood is no longer washed in and out with the tides. Instead, we stand at the shoreline and take in the full beauty of the sea, recognizing that our self—spirit—is one with that vast ocean.

My infertility patients in particular find peace of mind in nonidentification. These are women whose emotional ups and downs can last for years. They are liberated by the realization that they can *have* their anxiety and grief, but they are *not* their anxiety and grief. The same liberation is possible for women going through divorce, job loss, cancer, chronic pain or illness, the death of a loved one, or a difficult menopausal transition.

Reaching Out

Life crises are often crises of faith. The women who come to our Mind-Body Center for Women's Health are usually in trouble—mostly physical, but almost always emotional and spiritual, as well. While serious illness is itself traumatic, it often accompanies traumatic life events—a parent's ongoing illness, marital disruption, a child's behavior problems, severe work pressures, family tensions, or, even worse, a combination of these problems. At the nadir of these crises—the parent dies, the family tensions erupt, the marriage dissolves, the diagnosis is dire—we may wonder about God or spirit. In our private thoughts, we ask, "Is the Almighty rebuking me?" If so, our concept of a punitive deity can itself cause us to remove ourselves even further from belief and prayer. Just as alienating is the thought, "Does the Almighty care, or even exist?" This crisis of faith commonly leads to long-term disillusionment. For many of us, it's either the beginning or the apex of our estrangement from spirituality.

What do we do in such circumstances? Barbara Nielsen counsels the women in our program to take a step back and ask the deeper questions. She never proselytizes them to become religious or spiritual. But she does encourage them to find out whether disenchantment is their root belief or their defense against hurt. They can accomplish this by reaching out to a spiritual community to make the deeper investigation. Here, from a recent conversation, is how Barbara characterized the nature of this effort:

> They hold to the idea that God is uninvolved in my life. They think, "I've got that nailed down, I think that's probably the way it really is." But I've seen that change when people introspect, when they go into their inner selves. A shift happens and they say, "You know, that doesn't really resonate at a deep level with me. I'm going to look further. I'm going to explore and see what other people in my religious community think. I'm going to go through the

rituals, and see whether I feel the presence of God or whether I still feel that He is uninvolved." You can test out your belief—or your disbelief—in a spiritual community where you're involved in supportive relationships, service to others, ritual, and dialogue.

You may even enlist the aid of one person—a minister, priest, rabbi, imam, pastoral counselor, meditation teacher, guru, or healer—to help you work through your spiritual crisis. (Don't pick anyone who presses you to adopt their views. Reach out to those willing to honor your choices.) The process may lead you to substantially redefine your most basic spiritual assumptions. Barbara Nielsen calls this person a "spiritual director," and she credits such an individual with guiding her through a divorce after thirty-six years of marriage.

Barbara's spiritual director helped her "make sure I had done everything I could to make it work, so in the final analysis I knew it was spirit's will that the marriage end." He enabled her to accept that the marriage had not been a dreadful wrong turn in her life's path, but an integral part of her growth process. Their work together was not about "cursing him out, saying what a dreadful person he was, and of course I'm so righteous." Rather, it was "an issue of my soul's development . . . exploring the divine purpose in both the marriage *and* the divorce."

Whether you seek a "spiritual director," involvement in a spiritual community, or even just a deep-going dialogue with a good friend, reaching out is both a means and an end in your quest for inner peace in the midst of faith-challenging life crises.

Reaching out should not be narrowly defined as help-seeking. Service to others in our communities—the needy, those without resources, friends or acquaintances in trouble—is also a form of reaching out. Moreover, helping with an open heart is as emotionally and spiritually nurturing to ourselves as it is to those we help.

In his marvelous book *The Healing Power of Doing Good*, investigator Allan Luks documents the benefits people receive when they engage in "selfless" acts of caring. In a survey of almost 3,300 volunteers, Luks found that 95 percent of the respondents reported some "feel-good" sensations during or after their helping activities, and 90 percent of them rated their health as better than others their age. "The [helping] process can be effective to some degree for virtually every sort of human ill," writes Luks. "Regular helping of others can diminish the effects of disabling chronic pain and lessen the symptoms of physical distress. And it can ease the tension of able-bodied people who are overworked and living in stressful times."

Not that we should help others primarily because of the benefits we reap—that *would* be selfish in a twisted way. Rather, we can recognize that helping establishes a relationship with healing effects on both the giving and receiving side. But, you may ask, if I try to give more won't I deplete myself spiritually and physically? Wouldn't this be the opposite of self-nurture?

The solution is to distinguish between self-sacrifice driven by a need for approval versus service from the heart. In their book *How Can I Help?*, Ram Dass and Paul Gorman explain:

> Our work to move beyond separateness may also strengthen our sense of abundance. We feel like we need less because we're coming to see just how much we'll always have access to. We don't have to ration our helping acts quite so carefully. We needn't constantly measure just how much we'll be able to offer before we get depleted. We don't have to feel as if we are sacrificing by giving. Beyond separateness, service replenishes . . .

As Ram Dass and Gorman continue this passage, they capture how reaching out to help is spiritual sustenance when it's an expression of our connectedness to other sentient beings in our world:

> In turn, our helping actions will be less directed by the ego's personal agenda and need for constant reassurance. We won't be entering into service so much to gain intimacy, purpose, a sense of usefulness, and so on. We don't need to go anywhere special to attain these. They're in us already and available all around, simply as we understand our interrelatedness with all things. Our service, then, is less a function of personal motive and more an expression of spontaneous, appropriate caring.

Letting Go

Most of us have heard of the serenity prayer, which is so popular in 12-step recovery groups: "God, grant me the serenity to accept the things

I cannot change, the courage to change the things I can, and the wisdom to know the difference." Written by theologian Reinhold Niebuhr in the first half of the twentieth century, it's become a familiar phrase at this century's turn. But it has become part of the cultural lexicon for good reason. It contains a bit of wisdom few of us have been able to fully integrate into our lives, though we know we need to. Why is the serenity prayer so easy to recite but so hard to adopt?

For women, the answer is clear. We're currently being asked to be good wives, super-mothers, vibrant specimens of bodily perfection, and thriving career women, without letting any of these juggling balls tumble to the ground. That requires a fabulous capacity for control, and indeed, our culture pushes control as the great virtue women should embody. As long as we *do the right things,* the magazines and talk shows tell us, we can have the perfect marriages, families, bodies, careers. There's always a new technique—whether it's a sex technique, a parenting technique, an exercise technique, a diet technique, or a getting-ahead technique—that will lead, as in a simple math equation, from effort to outcome.

Many women suffer from low self-esteem precisely because they're disillusioned with themselves for not exerting enough control. Whenever we're unable to achieve a goal, we assume we either misapplied or neglected to do the *technique* we were told was the singular path to success and happiness. This leads us to feel perenially out of control, and guilty to boot—a frequent condition among the women I work with, no matter what the nature of their physical or emotional complaint.

Of course, we genuinely need a sense of control over our work, relationships, and health. Research by social psychologist Suzanne C. Ouellette, among others, has shown that people with confidence in their own ability to take charge of events are more able to resist stress-related illnesses. But here's the paradox: When we start buying into the belief that we should have *near-total* control over every facet of our lives, we've swallowed a delusion, which only makes us feel increasingly helpless. That's when the serenity prayer is so helpful: We need the utmost discernment to know where and when to exert control, and where and when to let go.

Given our cultural training, the letting go part is usually hardest, but it's the phase of coping that leads us toward the spiritual realm. Once we relinquish control, recognizing that we've done all we can to raise our kids properly, jump-start our careers, battle an illness, help a friend in trouble, put our creative works out in the world, prevent breast cancer, earn enough money, have a child, or make the marriage work, we can only "turn over" the outcome to some force beyond our reckoning.

Letting go is a difficult but rewarding art. It represents the healthiest kind of surrender—not giving *up*, but giving *in* to a higher power after we've put heart and soul into an arduous struggle or cherished endeavor. Over our life spans, and sometimes from month to month, we must alternate between control and letting go, in what amounts to a balancing act on the high wire between willful action and serene acceptance.

This balancing act was captured by Ken Wilber in his book *Grace and Grit*, which chronicles his and his wife Treya's struggle after she was diagnosed with metastatic breast cancer a mere ten days after they exchanged marital vows. Treya died five years later, and though the couple shared horrific lows as they fought her cancer, they also experienced exultant highs and a deepening of their commitment both to each other and to spiritual practice. Here is how Ken captured the balancing act:

> In addition to learning how to take control and assume responsibility, a person also needs to learn when and how to let go, to surrender, to go with the flow and not resist or fight it. Letting go versus taking control—that is, of course, just another version of being versus doing, that primordial polarity of yin and yang that assumes a thousand different forms and is never exhausted. It is not that yin or yang is right, that being is better than doing—it's a question of finding the right balance, finding the natural harmony between yin and yang that the ancient Chinese called Tao. Finding that balance—between doing and being, controlling and allowing, resisting and opening, fighting and surrendering, willing and accepting—finding that balance became the central issue in Treya's confrontation with cancer . . .

One of my infertility patients, Becky, struck her own version of this balance with discernment and gritty determination. Her story may have resonance for any woman struggling to realize a dream. By the time Becky joined one of our weekend workshops, she and her husband Rob had already spent years in fertility treatment. She committed herself to the approaches she learned at our retreat, including a slow-down in physical activity, which some studies indicate may increase chances of conception. (She's an exercise freak, so this was no small feat). She also used cognitive restructuring, and began meditating forty-five minutes each morning and night—well beyond our recommendations. "Going to the retreat was a turning point," Becky told me. "A light bulb went off and I understood for the first time that a number of factors could affect my fertility, especially if I integrated them in a program and practiced them with discipline."

Becky also knew, however, that her efforts were no guarantee of success. She ran up against a universal dilemma: How do we accept that our intentionality, wholeheartedness, and hard work *matter,* even when they can't be counted on to bring our dreams to fruition? She found an answer in a book, *The Life We Are Given,* by holistic pioneers George Leonard and Michael Murphy, who explain their concept of "focused surrender." "This practice combines strongly imaging a desired outcome in the present tense, as if it was already happening or had happened, then totally surrendering to grace."

At first, Becky was more perplexed than convinced by the descriptions of focused surrender. Yet she was intuitively drawn to the concept, sensing that it was a key to her ability to resolve her infertility. But it required a critical shift in her usual way of doing things. "I've always believed that if you work hard and put your nose to the grindstone, things will work out," she said, noting that up until then her determined efforts to get pregnant simply had not worked. "I had to realize the limits of my control in this process. I can control X, Y, and Z, but at a certain point I had to have faith that I'd done everything possible, and now it was out of my hands."

Soon after our workshop, Becky went through an in vitro fertilization (IVF) procedure that was unsuccessful. But she kept her wits about her, beginning her practice of focused surrender as she prepared for another IVF cycle. For Becky, what had been an intriguing abstraction was now an avenue to her own inner wisdom.

"I finally recognized that total control of this [fertility quest] was an illusion," she commented. "You can set the table, that's how I see it now. You put the silverware in the right place, position the place mats, set out beautiful flowers, prepare the food. Then it's out of your hands. The wrong combination of people may sit down at the table and it's a disaster. But the fact remains that the table was beautifully set, and the disaster has nothing to do with you. That realization is hard to come by when you have a high need for control."

On emotional and spiritual levels, Becky's practice paid off during the next IVF cycle. On the day the embryos were to be transferred, her trusted fertility specialist was called away, and the substitute doctor cast a negative pall over the event: he derided the quality of the embryos he was about to place in her uterus. It could have been her cue to freak out, but she turned instead to focused surrender. "I thought, I've done everything they've asked of me, and everything I've asked of myself. Now I can only have faith that whatever happens is for the best." She remained unflappably calm despite the stress and uncertainty surrounding the IVF process.

The cycle succeeded: Becky has since given birth to twins, and she's convinced that her efforts—as well as her nonefforts—contributed to her joyous result. She recalls the days and weeks prior to her successful IVF procedure: "When I finally let go, it was like skydiving. I had such a sense of peace." Becky was reminded of a comment once made to her by an employer who'd taken over sole responsibility for supervising her job. "I was nervous about it, because with the prior arrangement I felt more secure. But he said to me, 'Becky, don't worry, I'll catch you in the palm of my hand.' That's what I think about focused surrender. What I went through was scary, but I had to believe I'd be caught in the palm of His hand."

The Spirit of Writing

You can use writing exercises to explore your spiritual beliefs, feelings, and intuitions. When we rush about like whirling dervishes just to get the items crossed off our daily lists, we may find ourselves asking, Where is my spiritual center? What do I believe? How can I honor my beliefs? What rituals have meaning for me? How can I live a life consistent with my ethical and spiritual values? Meditation and relaxation are ways to clean your slate for answers, but writing can be a sturdy vehicle for a penetrating exploration.

Julia Cameron refers often to the spiritual dimension of writing; it's one reason she recommends the daily practice of "morning pages" (see chapter 6). "It is impossible to write morning pages for any extended period of time without coming into contact with an unexpected inner power," writes Cameron. "Although I used them for many years before I realized this, the pages are a pathway to a strong and clear sense of self. They are a trail that we follow into our own interior, where we meet both our own creativity and our creator."

Although writing out whatever impulses, insights, images, or ideas that come to mind is therapeutic and can lead to spiritual awakenings, we can also confront our spiritual beliefs and help ourselves locate our spiritual center through directed writing exercises. I suggest the following:

1. Write about the worst experience you can remember from your childhood associated with organized religion or spirituality.

2. Write about the best experience you can remember from your childhood associated with organized religion or spirituality.

3. Write out your deepest thoughts and feelings about your concept of spirit or God.

4. Write out your vision of the spiritual life you imagine would bring you the greatest peace of mind, wholeness, and sense of connection to something beyond yourself. How would your life change? How would it remain similar? What rituals might you practice that you don't now? How would your ethics change? How would your relations to others and your concept of spirit change?

HEARING THE SOUL'S WHISPERS: NURTURE THE SELF/SPIRIT

We have formalized, ritualized ways to nurture self and spirit (which are one and the same), and we have ways so embedded in our routine existence that we may not even recognize them. Maybe it's because I was raised without organized religious ritual, but my orientation to spiritual self-nurture has been entirely through the latter—moments in my relations with others, my work, my family, and my connection to nature in which I feel, instinctively and fleetingly, that something beyond my usual mental grasp has been revealed, something ethereal, timeless, and magical.

If you are not drawn to organized religion, perhaps you can focus on these moments, as I have, as your primary path to spiritual self-nurture. If you are either involved or drawn to organized religion, deepening your ritual practice may be your primary path, but you can also deepen your awareness of the sacred in the interstices of your existence, what Thomas Moore calls "the re-enchantment of everyday life."

My own moments of spiritual consciousness have been associated not with extraordinary events, but rather the most ordinary ones. Recently, a few weeks after a hectic holiday season, my husband and daughter and I spent a Sunday afternoon hanging out. We put on some music and danced, and I felt that familiar, strong connection with my husband that I've had hundreds of times before, yet which I consider a spiritual moment. Nothing otherworldly, just the feeling that we understand each other so completely that we are, in some sense, one with each other. I often have similar experiences with my daughter, such as when she spontaneously kisses me—a purely unconditional love.

We rarely regard the spiritual dimension of work, but I've had many experiences in my professional life that touch the transcendent, such as when data from one of my studies confirms the value of mind-body medicine for women. But my most meaningful work experiences have been with patients. When a woman suffering with stress or PMS or infertility or cancer says, "I've gotten my life back," I feel that my purpose has been fulfilled. If I've helped to ease her confusion, isolation, and pain, I have all the spiritual satisfaction I need. I believe that such experiences are indeed spiritual, and they speak to another less popularly recognized aspect of spirituality. Namely, when we realize our calling in acts of creativity, caring, relatedness—whatever—we come close to that sense of oneness with the Absolute.

In his challenging book *The Soul's Code,* James Hillman reaches for a spirituality born of realizing our unique calling in the world. He uses the metaphor of the acorn: Every majestic oak tree had its destiny—its shape, form, and life span—written in a tiny acorn. Likewise, each of us has his or her destiny written in a defining image, one that precedes us and that we spend our lives trying to fulfill, whether or not we realize it.

Hillman's idea sits on the shoulders of a myth laid forth by Plato in his *Republic*. Here is Hillman's description of Plato's myth:

> The soul of each of us is given a unique daimon before we are born, and it has selected an image or pattern that we live on earth. This soul-companion, the daimon, guides us here; in the process of arrival, however, we forget all that took place and believe we come empty into this world. The daimon remembers what is in your image and belongs to your pattern, and therefore the daimon is the carrier of your destiny.

What I like about Hillman is how he takes this compelling but rather abstract idea and makes it practical. We can take specific steps to live out our destiny, so our lives are rich with meaning and our potential for wholeness is actualized. We can start, says Hillman, by reframing ideas about our psychology that leads to victimization (i.e., we were crippled in childhood and now we're consigned to a lifetime of emotional reparations). We should review our lives through a different set of glasses, through "ideas of calling, of soul, of daimon, of fate, of necessity." Hillman continues:

> Then, the myth implies, we must attend very carefully to childhood to catch early glimpses of the daimon in action, to grasp its intentions and not block its way. The rest of the practical implications swiftly unfold: (a) Recognize the call as a prime fact of human existence; (b) align life with it; (c) find the common sense to realize that accidents, including the heartache and the natural shocks the flesh is heir to, belong to the pattern of the image, are necessary to it, and help fulfill it.

Hillman's idea of the soul's code resonates with me and with many women who are my patients and friends. I know that from a very young age I had a clear conviction: I was going to help women. When I look back at the twists and turns of my early school days, college years, and postgraduate studies, I followed numerous threads in various directions, but I kept returning to women's well-being. If I had ignored this calling, I don't believe I would have made the same contributions in another field. Today, when my work expands or suceeds, even in the smallest ways, from the modest triumph of one patient to the publication of one paper, I have that momentary experience of rightness in myself and the world.

Thus, a self-nurturing spirituality is more than prayer, more than affirmations, more than ritual, more than joining a spiritual community. It may be all of these. But it also asks you to unearth your defining image, your calling, the acorn of your being. Once you do, it is the height of self-nurture to align yourself with that image, to complete that calling, to realize your singular destiny. Remember, however, to do so with a fierce and tender concern for yourself, your loved ones, and your own conception of the Divine.

Appendix

Beach Walk Meditation

Close your eyes and begin to turn your attention to your breathing. Notice how your stomach rises and falls with each breath. Breathe in through your nose and out through your mouth, taking slow, deep breaths. Your stomach rises as you breathe in and falls as you breathe out. As you inhale, count slowly in your mind from 1 to 4, and as you exhale, count from 4 to 1. Pause for a few seconds after you inhale, and pause again for a few seconds after you exhale.

Do a quick mental check of your whole body, from the top of your head all the way down to your toes. As you inhale, concentrate on any area where you feel muscle tension or pain. As you exhale, release that muscle tension, your stomach rising as you breathe in and falling as you breathe out. Continue breathing slowly and deeply. Your stomach rises as you breathe in and falls as you breathe out. Notice how cool the air is as you breathe in through your nose and how warm it is as you breathe out through your mouth.

Imagine yourself at the top of a flight of stairs. At the bottom of the stairs is a beautiful beach with fine, white sand and sparkling blue water. As you stand at the top of the stairs, notice the beauty of the sand and the water and the clear blue sky. There are twenty steps between you and the beach. Very slowly, start to walk down the steps. Walk down the first step and the second step and the third step, then pause for a moment and look out over the beach. Feel the sun against your shoulders. Take a fourth step and a fifth step and a sixth step and a seventh step, then pause again. Take a slow, deep breath and look out over the beach and the sand and the water.

Take an eighth step and a ninth step and a tenth step. Now you're halfway down the stairs. Feel the sun against your shoulders. Listen to the roar of the ocean and smell the salt air; feel some sand beneath your feet. Take an eleventh step and a twelfth step and a thirteenth step and a fourteenth step. Pause again. You're closer to the beach now, so the sound of the ocean is a little louder, and you can feel the sun against your shoulders, and you can hear the waves breaking against the sand.

Take a fifteenth step and a sixteenth step and a seventeenth step. You're almost at the beach now, and you can feel the sun and smell the salt air, and feel more sand under you feet. Take an eighteenth step and a nineteenth step and a twentieth step onto the sand. Now you're standing on the beach, and you pause for just a second and take a nice, slow, deep breath. Breathe in the warm salty air. Then very slowly start to walk toward the water, feeling the warm sand under your feet and the sun against your back, hearing the water, and smelling the salt air. Walk very, very slowly toward the water. When you get close to the water, stand there for a while, watching the waves coming in and going out. Enjoy the solitude and the peace.

After a few moments, you might choose to start walking up the beach. You might walk close to the water, so you walk in the wet sand, or you might walk a little higher up where the sand is dry and warm. As you slowly stroll the beach, look out over the horizon at the white-crested waves. Notice the seagulls flying overhead. You might look down at your feet and notice the sand and the shells and the little bits of seaweed.

Stop and look out over the water and take a slow, deep breath of the fresh, quiet air. Then turn around and start to walk back down the beach, walking very slowly, noticing the shells and the water and the sand and the sun.

You might sit down in the sand, noticing how soft and warm the sand is beneath you. Look out over the water, noticing the sun reflecting against the water, watching the waves flowing in and going out.

After a while, as your time at the beach draws to an end, stand up and look out over the beach. Take some slow, deep breaths, breathing in the warm salty air, absorbing the beauty and the solitude of the beach and looking out as the waves flow in and out.

Take another slow, deep breath, then slowly turn around and start to walk toward the staircase, noticing the warm sand under your feet and the sun against your face. As you walk slowly toward the stairs, hear the ocean behind you and feel the sun in front of you. When you get to the bottom of the stairs, turn around and take one last look at the beach and the water. Take one last, slow, deep breath, then very slowly start to climb the stairs, one step at a time. Every once in a while, stop and turn around and look at the beach, then go back to climbing the stairs.

When you get to the top of the stairs, turn your attention to your breathing, noticing your stomach rising as you breathe in and falling as you breathe out, breathing in through your nose and out through your mouth, taking slow, deep breaths.

Now, count down from 10, one number for each breath, pausing for a few seconds after you inhale and after you exhale. When you reach 0, begin to pay attention to some of the sounds in the room. Become aware of where your body is. When you feel ready, slowly, slowly open your eyes, but keep your gaze lowered for a few minutes and just lie quietly, as you reacquaint yourself with the room.

MOUNTAIN STREAM MEDITATION

Seat yourself comfortably. (Do not lie down.) Close your eyes and slowly inhale and exhale. Beginning with your forehead, move down the length of your body, from your forehead to your eyes to your cheeks to your jaw to your mouth. As you inhale, concentrate on each different body part. As you exhale, let go of any muscle tension that may be there. Move all the way down from the top of your head to your toes, becoming aware and releasing any muscle tension you may have.

As you inhale, mentally count from 1 to 4, and as you exhale, count from 4 to 1. Make each breath as long and slow as possible. Pause for a second or two after you inhale, then exhale and pause again, slowing down your breathing.

Imagine yourself standing on a path in very thick, dark woods. As you stand there, notice lots of trees around you. Feel the soft pine needles beneath your feet. Start walking along the path and notice that you're twenty steps away from a mountain stream. Take the first step and notice the rustle of the wind through the trees. Take a second step and notice the pine needles beneath your feet. Take a third step and begin to hear the water along the rocks in the stream. Take a fourth step and fifth step, then stop and notice that it's getting a little lighter as you

approach the stream. But you're still in the woods, and you are still surrounded by many trees.

Take a sixth step, then a seventh step, noticing the trees and the moss
and the pine needles. Take an eighth step and a ninth step and a tenth
step, then stop and notice that the sound of the water is louder. As you
move closer to the stream, you begin to see more light between the trees.
You're still in the woods but you're becoming more aware of the nearby
mountain stream. Take an eleventh step and a twelfth step. You can hear
the water more clearly. Take a thirteenth step and a fourteenth step.
You're starting to come out of the woods now. The trees are farther
apart, and it's lighter, and the sound of the water is getting louder.

Take a fifteenth step and a sixteenth step and a seventeenth step. Notice that the ground beneath you is feeling spongier, and more light is
filtering through the trees, and the sound of the water is getting louder
as you walk. You take an eighteenth step and a nineteenth step and the
last, twentieth, step. Now the stream is in front of you. Stand quietly for
a few moments and notice the stream. Notice what you can see, what
you can hear, and what you can feel.

You might sit down on a rock by the stream and look into the water,
being aware of what you can see in the water, of the wind against
your cheeks, of the sound of the water, the sound of nearby birds.
Sit quietly on the rock as you absorb the peace and the beauty of your
surroundings.

Stand up and walk to where the water cascades down in a small
waterfall. Feel the spray of the water as it splashes down and hear the
sound of the water as it flows over the rocks. Stand still and enjoy the serenity. Breathe in the fresh air and the quiet and the peace.

Walk along the stream for a few feet, looking at different patterns of
water around the rocks. Put your hand in the water and feel how cold it
is. Sit and watch and listen and feel.

As the time for your visit to the stream draws to an end, spend another minute or two standing quietly, breathing in the peace and serenity and beauty. Listen to the water and feel the breeze on your face
and in your hair.

As you turn around and go back to the beginning of the path, carry
with you a sense of beauty and peace from the stream. Take one last
look, breathing slowly and deeply. Then turn around and take your first
step along the path. Take a second step, and pause and listen to the

water. Take a third step, then a fourth step, and a fifth step as you start to get into the woods. Although now you are surrounded by more trees, you can still hear the stream. You can still feel the breeze from the water. You take a sixth step and a seventh step and an eighth step, and now you're farther along the path. You can feel the pine needles under your feet, and it's getting a little darker as you move deeper into the woods. Take a ninth step and a tenth step and you're halfway along the path now. Turn around; you can just barely see the stream. The trees are thicker in this part of the forest. You can feel the pine needles beneath your feet, and you can smell the pine cones.

Take an eleventh step and a twelfth step and a thirteenth step. Now stop for a moment. You can still hear the stream, but it's a little fainter. Take a fourteenth step and a fifteenth step. You're more aware of the quiet of the woods, of the trees around you, of pine needles beneath your feet. Take a sixteenth step and a seventeenth step. You can barely hear the stream behind you, but you carry part of it with you. Take an eighteenth step and a nineteenth step and a twentieth step. Now, with your eyes still closed, return to noticing your breath. Become aware of your stomach rising as you breathe in and falling as you breathe out.

As you inhale, silently count from 1 to 4. As you exhale, reverse the count, from 4 to 1. Breathe in and out slowly for a few more minutes.

As the time for this relaxation comes to an end, begin to become aware of your surroundings, where you are seated, what sounds you are hearing. When you feel ready, slowly open your eyes and keep your gaze lowered for a few minutes. When you feel ready, look up and slowly get out of your chair.

RELAXATION AUDIOTAPES YOU CAN ORDER

The following resource audiotapes are available through the Mind/Body Medical Clinic, Attn: Tapes, 110 Francis Street, Suite 1A, Boston, MA 02215 (617) 632-9530 and press 0.

Each tape is $10; please make checks payable to BIDMC. Tapes are non-refundable. For checks drawn on banks outside the United States, please add an additional $10 per tape (U.S. dollars only).

Basic Relaxation Exercise/Mindfulness Meditation (female voice)
Side 1 (20 minutes): This side introduces a basic relaxation sequence to help you elicit the relaxation response, including some of the key elements,

such as breath awareness, body scan relaxation, and the use of a focus word. Specific instructions throughout the tape aid in the initial development of your experience of the relaxation response.

Side 2 (20 minutes): This side offers instruction on awareness, or "mindfulness," of sensations, thoughts, and sounds. It also introduces breath and awareness as "primary tools" that enable you to integrate the relaxation response into daily activities. This side has fewer instructions, allowing you to further develop your relaxation response techniques.

Basic Relaxation Response Exercise (male voice)

Side 1 (20 minutes): This tape is very similar to the other Basic Relaxation tape; however, this one features a male voice. It also introduces breath awareness and body scan relaxation.

Side 2 (45 minutes): Side 2 offers frequent pauses to allow you to practice techniques that elicit the relaxation response.

Advanced Relaxation Response (female voice)

Side 1 (30 minutes): This side guides you through a body scan and relaxation, leading you into a relaxation response through awareness of your heart and repetition of your focus word. This tape has frequent pauses to encourage you to practice and develop ways of bringing forth the relaxation response on your own.

Side 2 (50 minutes): Side 2 reinforces basic skills and also guides you through a stretching routine and a series of images for healing.

A Gift of Relaxation/Garden of Your Mind (female voice)

Side 1, *Gift of Relaxation* (20 minutes): This side focuses on introducing the basic steps of eliciting the relaxation response. You are quietly guided through body scan relaxation exercises and some simple deep breathing techniques, which are intended to heighten your awareness and enable you to deepen your experience of the relaxation response. The tape ends with positive affirmations, encouraging you to feel good about yourself and be proud of your experience.

Side 2, *Garden of Your Mind* (20 minutes): This creative mental imagery exercise begins with body scan relaxation and breath awareness components and incorporates imagery of a lovely garden, one that you have visited in your past or one that you create in your own mind. The tape ends with positive self-statements and encouragement.

Self-Empathy/Nurturing Change (female voice)

Side 1 (20 minutes): Accompanied by peaceful and rhythmic music, this side uses guided meditation useful to counter anxiety. Breath focus is used to support nonjudging awareness followed by progressive body relaxation. Self-empathy becomes the focus, guided by self-awareness and steps leading to one's intention for happiness.

Side 2 (18 minutes): This side uses music and guided meditation to enhance self-awareness, acceptance, and control through breathing, contemplation, and intentions for greater physical and emotional well-being.

Rest in Gratitude/Healing Light (female voice)

Side 1 (19 minutes): This side uses guided imagery that invites you through a gentle body scan accompanied by soft music. You are asked to focus on and develop an awareness of various parts of your body. This is a very soothing and restful way to elicit the relaxation response and develop nonjudgmental, focused awareness.

Side 2 (19 minutes): This side uses breath awareness and ocean sounds and guides you to focus on a soothing, healing light, emphasizing rest and healing. The ocean sounds are used as background during a time of quiet, focused, deep relaxation.

Relaxation Exercises I and II (female voice)

Side 1 (20 minutes): This side introduces a basic relaxation sequence based on progressive muscle relaxation to help you elicit the relaxation response. Specific instructions throughout the tape aid in the initial development of your experience and the tape ends with a peaceful brief visualization.

Side 2 (14 minutes): This side guides you through a body scan and relaxation, leading you into elicitation of the relaxation response through awareness of gently releasing tension throughout your body. The tape ends with a peaceful brief visualization.

Relaxation Exercise/Mountain Stream Mental Imagery (female voice)

Side 1 (20 minutes): This side gently guides you through a series of breathing techniques leading into body scan relaxation. Its purpose is to alleviate tension from each body part and allows you to practice breathing awareness. This side of the tape also includes a word-focus exercise.

Side 2 (20 minutes): Side 2 offers you creative imagery acting as a tour guide on a walk through a forest to a mountain stream, allowing you to escape and become aware of and focus on your senses.

Tuning In to Your Body, Tuning Up Your Mind (female voice)

Side 1 (30 minutes): This side guides you through chair and standing exercises. The exercises emphasize releasing physical tension, loosening joints, and realigning posture. The practice session encourages elicitation of the relaxation response through mindfulness.

Side 2 (30 minutes): This side offers instruction in floor exercises found in *The Wellness Book*. It includes special instruction in diaphragmatic breathing and gives guidance for using your breath to enhance your exercise practice. This side ends with a deep relaxation. A diagram is included.

An Introduction to the Relaxation Response/A Special Time for You (female voice)

Side 1 (20 minutes): Side 1 introduces the practice of the relaxation response. It offers instruction in diaphragmatic breathing and the release of physical tension. The tape guides your practice by focusing on the breath, a word or phrase, and the creative imagination of a safe place. (This tape is suitable for someone learning the relaxation response.)

Side 2 (20 minutes): This side gives gentle guidance in the practice of the relaxation response using imagery, body scan relaxation, and breath focus. The tape emphasizes the use of the breath and the practice of nonjudging awareness to decrease tension and to soothe physical discomfort.

Extended Relaxation Exercise/Beach Walk Mental Imagery (female voice)

Side 1 (40 minutes): Side 1 focuses on relaxation exercises, including a long body scan relaxation to relieve tension from every body part. It then leads you through visualization of taking a warm, comfortable bath. The guidance in this tape is very specific, making it quite easy to follow. You may find this longer side useful during medical, surgical, or dental procedures.

Side 2 (20 minutes): Side 2 directs you through a series of breath and other relaxation exercises that elicit the relaxation response followed by a guided imagery exercise of exploring a sandy beach on a magnificent summer day. (This differs from the ocean waves tape because there are no wave sounds in the background.)

Guided Visualization with Ocean Sounds/Breath and Body Awareness (female voice)

Side 1 (24 minutes): Side 1 is a guided body scan relaxation. It incorporates guided visualization of a sandy ocean beach, enhanced by the soothing ocean sounds in the background.

Side 2 (30 minutes): Side 2 leads you through a series of stretching exercises done in a sitting position. These stretches will encourage a peaceful state of relaxation, awareness, and the elicitation of the relaxation response. This side of the tape does not use ocean wave sounds.

Exercise and the Relaxation Response (male voice)

Side 1 (31 minutes): This side offers instruction on how to elicit the relaxation response while exercising. This tape serves as a verbal guide to help you combine the practices of exercise and the relaxation response to enhance your mental health as you improve your physical fitness.

Side 2 (31 minutes): This side has nondistracting music that fills the silence and is helpful once instruction from the first side is no longer needed.

Positive Affirmations and Visualization in Weight Loss (female voice)

Side 1 (13 minutes): Accompanied by soft music, side 1 uses positive affirmations to enhance positive thinking when you are dealing with food issues and body image.

Side 2 (11 minutes): This tape uses guided imagery that invites you through a gentle body scan also accompanied by soft music and nature sounds. The tape ends with positive affirmations encouraging you to gain acceptance of where you are and who you are, thereby creating the potential for change and learning to love the body you have.

Safe Place/Pain Visualization (female voice)

Side 1 (22 minutes): This side offers a guided meditation with progressive muscle relaxation and visualization of a safe place for patients with chronic pain. This tape will be helpful for those who might experience anxiety or feelings of vulnerability during the relaxation response process.

Side 2 (22 minutes): This side guides you through an advanced meditation with body sweeps of progressive relaxation and visualization of pain imagery. This is potentially a very helpful exercise for pain control.

Basic Yoga Stretching Exercises/Stretching and Balancing Exercises (female voice)

Side 1 (20 minutes): Side 1 encourages you to focus on energizing your body. You are guided through a series of gentle stretches and relaxation exercises to reinforce diaphragmatic breathing. The moderate pace allows ample time for you to participate in the activities to enhance your relaxation response experience. Side 1 ends in an exercise to elicit the relaxation response.

Side 2 (20 minutes): Side 2 encourages you to follow along in a gentle, slow-paced routine of stretching and movement awareness. Its purpose is to decrease muscular tension and elicit the relaxation response.

Relaxation Exercises for Students—Tape 1 (female voice)
Special Place / Worries in a Box / Music Relaxation 1 and 2 / Mountain Meditation / Melting the Dime Spot (pain reduction).

Relaxation Exercises for Students—Tape 2 (female and male voices)
Breath Focus Relaxation / Muscle Relaxation / Beach Walk / Garden Walk.

Selected Bibliography

Achterberg, Jeanne. *Imagery in Healing.* Boston: New Science Library, 1985.
———, Barbara Dossey, and Leslie Kolkmeier. *Rituals of Healing: Using Imagery for Health and Wellness.* New York: Bantam Books, 1994.
Ban Breathnach, Sarah. *Simple Abundance: A Daybook of Comfort and Joy.* New York: Warner Books, 1997.
Beck, Martha. *Breaking Point: Why Women Fall Apart and How They Can Re-create Their Lives.* New York: Times Books, 1997.
Benson, Herbert, and Miriam Klipper. *The Relaxation Response.* New York: Avon, 1976.
———, with Marg Stark. *Timeless Healing: The Power and Biology of Belief.* New York: Scribner, 1996.
Borysenko, Joan. *Minding the Body, Mending the Mind.* Reading, MA: Addison-Wesley, 1987.
———. *A Woman's Book of Life: The Biology, Psychology, and Spirituality of the Feminine Life Cycle.* New York: Putnam, 1997.
Chernin, Kim. *Hungry Self: Women, Eating, and Identity.* New York: Times Books, 1985.
Domar, Alice, and Henry Dreher. *Healing Mind, Healthy Woman: Using the Mind-Body Connection to Manage Stress and Take Control of Your Life.* New York: Delacorte, 1997.
Dossey, Larry. *Healing Words: The Power of Prayer and the Practice of Medicine.* New York: Harper Collins, 1993.
Dreher, Henry. *The Immune Power Personality: 7 Traits You Can Develop to Stay Healthy.* New York: Dutton Books, 1995.
Gilligan, Carol. *In a Different Voice: Psychological Theory and Women's Development.* Cambridge, MA: Harvard University Press, 1982.
Goleman, Daniel, ed. *Healing Emotions: Conversations with the Dalai Lama on Mindfulness, Emotions, and Health.* Boston: Shambhala Publications, 1997.

Gordon, Lynn. *52 Silly Things to Do When You're Blue.* San Francisco: Chronicle Books, 1994.

Kabat-Zinn, Jon. *Full Catastrophe Living: Using the Wisdom of Your Body and Mind to Face Stress, Pain, and Fear.* New York: Delacorte, 1991.

————. *Wherever You Go, There You Are.* New York: Hyperion, 1994.

————. *Everyday Blessings: The Inner Work of Mindful Parenting.* New York: Hyperion, 1998.

Lerner, Harriet. *The Dance of Anger: A Woman's Guide to Changing the Patterns of Intimate Relationships.* New York: Harper and Row, 1985.

————. *The Dance of Intimacy: A Woman's Guide to Courageous Acts of Change in Key Relationships.* New York: Harper and Row, 1989.

Levine, Stephen. *Healing into Life and Death.* New York: Anchor Books, 1987.

————. *Guided Meditations, Explorations, and Healings.* New York: Anchor Books, 1991.

Lindbergh, Anne Morrow. *Gift from the Sea.* New York: Pantheon, 1991.

Luks, Allan, with Peggy Payne. *The Healing Power of Doing Good.* New York: Fawcett Columbine, 1992.

Northrup, Christiane. *Women's Bodies, Women's Wisdom: Creating Physical and Emotional Health and Healing.* 2nd Edition. New York: Bantam Books, 1998.

Ornish, Dean. *Love and Survival: The Scientific Basis for the Healing Power of Intimacy.* New York: HarperCollins, 1998.

Ornstein, Robert, and David Sobel. *Healthy Pleasures.* Reading, MA: Addison-Wesley, 1989.

Pennebaker, James. *Opening Up: The Healing Power of Expressing Emotions.* New York: Guilford Press, 1997.

Remen, Rachel Naomi. *Kitchen Table Wisdom: Stories That Heal.* New York: Riverhead, 1996.

Rodin, Judith. *Body Traps: Breaking the Binds That Keep You from Feeling Good.* New York: William Morrow, 1992.

Scarf, Maggie. *Intimate Worlds: Life Inside the Family.* New York: Random House, 1995.

————. *Intimate Partners: Patterns in Love and Marriage.* New York: Ballantine, 1996.

Steinem, Gloria. *Revolution from Within: A Book of Self-esteem.* Boston: Little, Brown. 1993.

Vanzant, Iyanla. *One Day, My Soul Just Opened Up.* New York: Fireside, 1998.

————. *Yesterday, I Cried.* New York: Simon & Schuster, 1999.

Vienne, Veronique, and Erica Lennard. *The Art of Doing Nothing: Simple Ways to Make Time for Yourself.* New York: Clarkson Potter, 1998.

Index